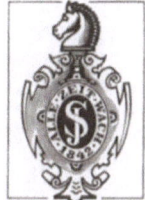

Current Concepts in Pediatric Radiology

Edited by O. Eklöf

With Contributions of
R. Astley, V. Boston, D. Brockwell, S. Cadranel, A. R. Chrispin
M. Cremer, N. Cremer, B. J. Cremin, C. Fauré, H. Fendel, A. Giedion
B. R. Girdany, G. B. C. Harris, M. Hassan, M. A. Lassrich, W. Porstmann
A. K. Poznanski, P. Rodesch, F. N. Silverman, G. Theander

With 165 Figures (265 Separate Illustrations)

Springer International 1977

Current Diagnostic Pediatrics, Volume 1

Series Editor:
Dr. Alan R. Chrispin
The Hospital for Sick Children,
X-Ray Department
Great Ormond Street
London WC 1 N 3JH
England

Volume Editor:
Dr. Ole Eklöf
Röntgenavdelingen, Barnkliniken
Karolinska Sjukhuset
10401 Stockholm 60
Sweden

ISBN-13: 978-3-540-08279-8   e-ISBN-13: 978-1-4471-1288-4
DOI: 10.1007/978-1-4471-1288-4

Library of Congress Cataloging in Publication Data. Main entry under title: Current concepts in pediatric radiology. (Current diagnostic pediatrics; v. 1) "Based on the lectures given at the First International Post-Graduate Course presented by the Swedish Society of Pediatric Radiology in May 1976." Includes bibliographical references and indes. 1. Pediatric radiology-Congress. I. Eklöf, Ole, 1925 – II. Astley, Roy. III. Series. RJ51.R3C87   618.9'2007'572
77-21744

Printing and bookbinding: Brühlsche Universitätsdruckerei, Lahn-Giessen
2123/3140-543210

Preface

The first radiological examination of an infant was reported as early as 1896. This was the prelude to a tremendous amount of pioneer work which was accomplished in the following decades. Interaction of increasing experience, technical improvement and new therapeutic achievement led to the present status of pediatric radiology. In almost any investigation and evaluation of childhood disease, pediatric radiology has a cardinal role.

The establishment of the European Society of Pediatric Radiology in 1963, and the start of the journal *Pediatric Radiology* 10 years later, have created international platforms for the circulation of rapidly accumulating knowledge. Both ventures have helped to underpin high educational standards in the specialty. In many countries national post-graduate courses have contributed quite admirably to favourable trends. More than ever, today medicine is an international science: medical training on an international level has therefore come to stay. This results in a more rapid dissemination of "Current Concepts in Pediatric Radiology" among all those devoted to this fascinating branch of radiology.

This book, mainly based on the lectures given at the First International Post-Graduate Course sponsored by the Swedish Society of Pediatric Radiology in May 1976, presents the contributions of the distinguished guest speakers on selected topics.

It is my belief, as Editor, that this volume will serve as a permanent record and provide interesting reading for those who were unable to attend. For those who had the chance of participating in this meeting the volume will be a useful written statement of the information presented.

Stockholm, September 1977   OLE EKLÖF

Contents

Contents

List of Authors

Dr. R. Astley
Deparment of Radiology
The Children's Hospital
Birmingham, B16 8ET, England

Dr. S. Cadranel
Gastro-enterological Unit
Departement Radiologie Pediatrique
Hôpital Saint-Pierre
Rue Haute, 322
B-1000 Bruxelles

Dr. A. R. Chrispin
The Hospital for Sick Children
X-Ray Department
Great Ormond Street
London, W.C. 1N 3JH, England

Dr. M. Cremer
Department of Gastro-enterology
Hôpital Universitaire Brugmann
B-1000 Bruxelles

Dr. N. Cremer
Departement Radiologie Pediatrique
Hôpital Saint-Pierre
Rue Haute, 322
B-1000 Bruxelles

Prof. B. J. Cremin
Dr. V. Boston
Dr. D. Brockwell
University of Cape Town
Department of Radiology
Groote Schuur Hospital
Observatory, 7925, South Africa

Dr. C. Fauré
Service de Radiologie
Hôpital Trousseau
8-28 avenue de Docteur-Arnold-Netter
F-75571 Paris Cedex 12

Dr. Fendel
Kinderklinik der Universität
München im Dr. von Haunerschen
Kinderspital
Lindwurmstraße 4
D-8000 München 2

Prof. Dr. A. Giedion
Abt. Radiologie
Kinderspital Zürich
Steinwiesstraße 75
CH-8032 Zürich

Dr. B. R. Girdany
University of Pittsburgh
School of Medicine
Department of Radiology
Pittsburgh, PA 15261, USA

Dr. G. B. C. Harris
The Children's Hospital Medical
Center
300 Longwood Avenue
Boston, Massachusetts 02115, USA

Dr. A. K. Poznanski
Division of Pediatric Radiology
C.S. Mott Children's Hospital
Univ. of Michigan Medical Center
Ann Arbor, Michigan 48101, USA

Dr. M. Hassan
Service de Radiologie
Hôpital Saint-Vincent-de-Paul
74, avenue Denfert-Rochereau
F-75014 Paris

Dr. P. Rodesch
Gastro-enterological Unit
Department Radiologie Pediatrique
Hôpital Saint-Pierre
Rue Haute, 322
B-1000 Bruxelles

Prof. Dr. M. A. Lassrich
Universitäts-Kinderklinik
Röntgenabteilung
Martinistr. 52
D-2000 Hamburg 20

Dr. F. N. Silverman
Department of Radiology
Stanford University Medical Center
Stanford, California 94305, USA

Prof. Dr. Sc. med. W. Porstmann
Abt. für radio-vaskuläre Diagnostik
Humboldt-Univ. zu Berlin
Schumannstr. 20—21
DDR-104 Berlin

Dr. G. Theander
Department of Radiology
Malmö Allmänna Sjukhus
S-214 01 Malmö

Radiology of Respiratory Distress in the Newborn

A "Gamut of Pattern" Approach

A. Giedion

1. Introduction

The following "primer" is adressed to colleagues with little experience in this field of neonatal radiology. The identification of typical patterns should be helpful in establishing a list of possible diagnoses (gamut); the final correct choice will usually be guided by the clinical circumstances. Obviously, only an intimate knowledge of physiology, pathophysiology and pathology of the newborn will enable the radiologist to reach a mature judgement. The interested reader is referred to several excellent books and numerous publications for a more extended study of this subject [1, 4, 34, 38, 41].

A first version of our somewhat primitive pattern-gamut approach was published 10 years ago [13] and summarized in the syllabus of the 18th (1975) San Francisco postgraduate course in diagnostic radiology [16]. This method has been, in our hands, particularly helpful for the instruction of our residents working in the newborn unit. Here, fast decisions have to be made at odd times, when an experienced interpreter of the radiologic findings may not be available.

The complex problem of congenital heart disease in the newborn will not be discussed in this paper, and you are referred to some recent publications [19, 22]. Only some implications on the pulmonary pattern, caused by congenital heart disease, will be mentioned. We should, however, keep in mind that a most severe example of congenital heart disease, e.g., transposition of the great vessels with little cross shunt, may have a normal chest, as opposed to a cyanotic baby with pulmonary congestion and an enlarged heart, caused by too high a hematocrit [13].

2. Preliminary Scan of the "Babygram"

Instead of a chest film we prefer, for our initial examination, a "babygram". Changes visible in the skeleton (e. g., syphilis, bone dysplasias), a ruptured spleen, a large liver in congenital heart disease etc., all conditions leading to "respiratory distress", may be recognized at a glance. Also film quality, artifacts, position of the diaphragm etc., have to be checked before concentrating on the chest.

2.1. The Main Types of Pattern to be Distinguished (Fig. 1)

Sometimes, even the decision whether or not a newborn chest is normal or abnormal may be difficult in view of transient normal but quite striking pulmonary patterns [29].

The White (Water Density) Chest (Table 1). Its recognition offers no problem. Obviously, the white chest is the normal radiological appearance before the first breath [11]. Only few of the many causes will be suspected on the evidence of a single film (Table 1). Some additional clinical facts, e.g., bloody foam from the airways or the knowledge of earlier films, showing the reticular granular pattern of hyaline membrane disease, may still allow the correct radiologic diagnosis. Although quite rare, the immediate recognition of a hydrothorax (Fig. 2) is even more urgent than that of a tension pneumothorax [12].

The Black (Air Density) Chest (Table 2). This group contains only two major diagnoses. Yet, just because these films are apparently typical, they have to be analyzed with particular care.

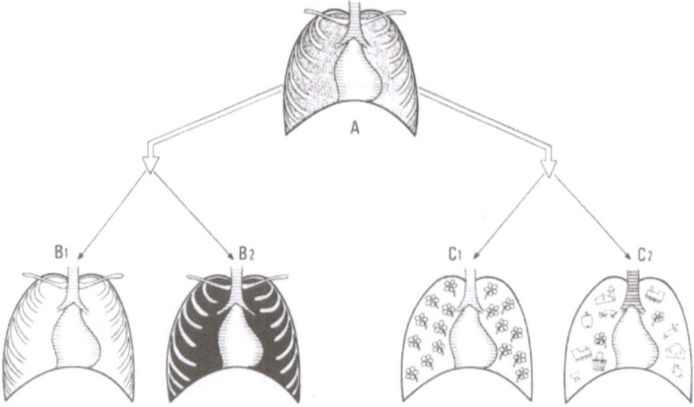

Fig. 1. Schematic drawing displaying the 5 basic "patterns" of the newborn chest. A = normal, Bl = "white" chest (water density), B2 = "black" chest (air density), Cl = regular pattern, C2 = irregular pattern

Table 1."White thorax" (water density) of the newborn

Pathogenesis	Cause/Disease
I. Atelectasis	Primary/Secondary > Surfactant (HMD) Hypoplastic lung
II. Alveoli filled or overdistended with fluid	Primary apnea Retention of alveolar fluid (Obstruction) Pulmonary edema Massive aspiration Alveolar hemorrhage Pneumonia
III. Displacement of pulmonary tissue (space-occupying mass)	Tumor (diaphragmatic, hernia)
IV. Pleural fluid	Hydro-chylo-hemato-infuso-urinothorax [11a, 12, 23, 35]

Table 2. Black thorax (air density) of the newborn

(Pseudo) pneumothorax
Alveolar emphysema (1st/2nd)
"Cysts"
(Oligemia)

Furthermore, a highly significant *tension pneumothorax* may be missed in the supine newborn, if only "free air" or displacement of the mediastinal structures is looked for. The "free air", sitting as a bubble on *top* of the lung, may just compress it and change its pattern (flattened—out lung). The "sharp edge sign" [32] is caused by the interface air/mediastinum as opposed to the normal interface lung/mediastinum, causing a more than usually sharp outline of heart and thymus. Both signs allow a preliminary diagnosis. The free substernal air may be demonstrated in a lateral chest film, horizontal beam, supine position of the baby [26]. In our hands, a-p views, the baby lying on its healthy side and with a horizontal beam, have been more diagnostic (Fig. 3).

The most deceiving picture of an *inflated intrathoracic stomach* (Fig. 4) illustrates the need for a careful examination even of seemingly "obvious" cases. Also large cysts, alveolar emphysema and skin-folds may be misinterpreted as pneumothorax (pseudopneumothorax, Table 3). The radiologically quite uniform appearance of *unilateral alveolar emphysema* may be caused by a variety of anatomical factors [21]. A few distinctive features are mentioned in Table 4. In this condition, the

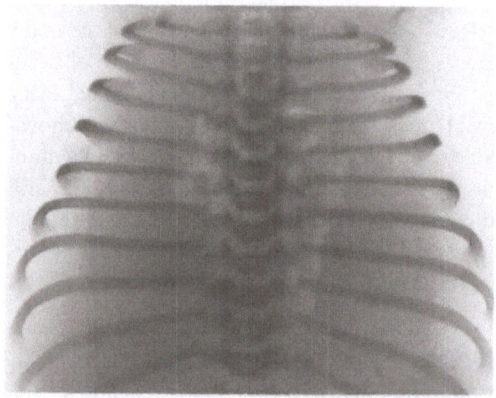

Fig. 2. Hydrothorax. Female 3 h old. Note expanded white chest. Some paraspinal air (artificial respiration). (From [12])

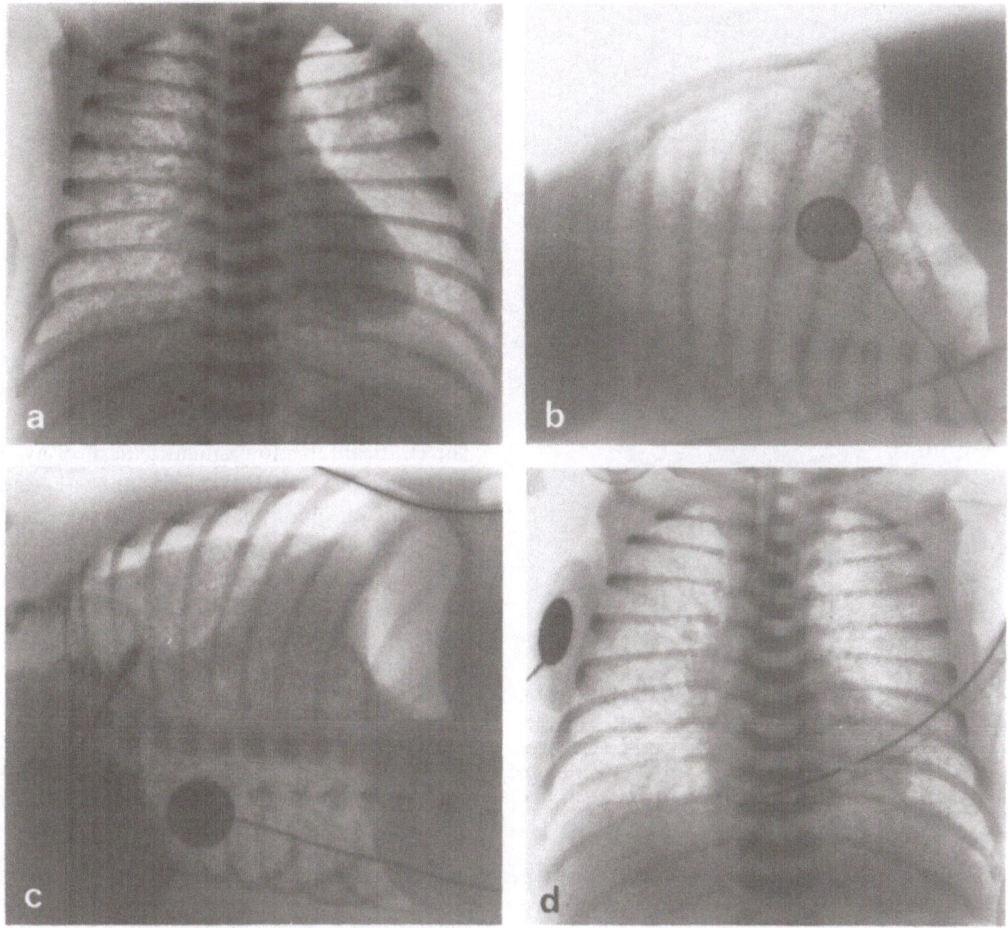

Fig. 3a–d. Female 2 days old. a) On right side typical miliary interstitial emphysema, which is similar, but lighter on left side (pattern change!). b) Lateral view, horizontal beam, with patient in supine position is inconclusive (no free air below sternum visible). c) A-p view, horizontal beam, patient lying on his healthy side, discloses large amount of air (tension pneumothorax). d) After successful treatment an identical pattern on both sides

involvement of all lobes on one side speaks against the most common idiopathic type, where the lower lobes are usually atelectatic. A few additional typical X-ray findings may offer valuable diagnostic clues: An esophagogram, e.g., may reveal a bronchogenic cyst, which can be missed even at operation with a subsequent unnecessary pneumonectomy [10] (Fig. 5). The radiologic work-up of alveolar emphysema should therefore include an esophagogram and possibly a preoperative bronchogram. In cases where a cardiovascular factor is suspected (Table 4) angiocardiography may be helpful. Finally, for correct longitudinal interpretation, the three phases of bronchial obstruction have to be understood by the radiologist (Fig. 6) [3, 8, 18].

The Regular Pattern (Table 5). The distinction of a (round) air space and a reticular-interstitial-nodular pattern (Fig. 7) is of course quite arbitrary and mainly didactic.

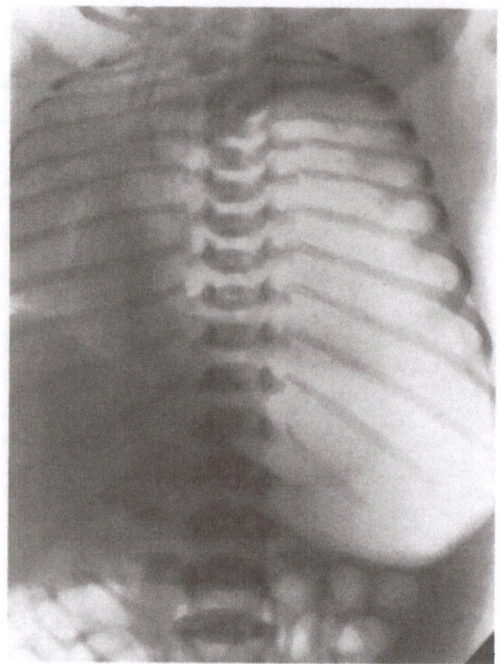

Fig. 4. Female, several hours old, intrathoracic stomach (large diaphragmatic hernia), simulating tension pneumothorax. Note defects in cervicothoracic spine, site of anterior meningomyelocele. (By courtesy of Dr. Bärlocher, Kinderspital St. Gallen)

Table 3. Pneumothorax of the newborn

Radiologic types

1. Asymptomatic
2. Classical tension
3. Atypical tension
4. Pseudo

The Round Air Space Pattern (Table 5A and Figs. 8 and 9). The main distinctive features between the various types is the changing ratio between "air holes" and the surrounding pulmonary framework.

The classical reticulo granular pattern of hyaline membrane disease (HMD) (Fig. 8a) has been observed also in pure pulmonary hemorrhage [25] and β-hemolytic streptococcal disease [3, 38a, 40]. The suggestion of the latter possibility by the radiologist might be life-saving to the patient. HMD disease of course presents radiologically the whole spectrum from near normal to a white chest. *Miliary interstitial pulmonary emphysema* (Fig. 8b,c) has been recognized only recently [6, 24]. Artificial respiration with sometimes considerable peak pressures has contributed to its in-

Table 4. Radiologic differential diagnosis of some types of unilateral alveolar emphysema[a]

	Distribution	Radiologic hint	Cause
Idiopathic lobar emphysema	Usually upper and/or middle lobe	Atelectatic lower lobe	Majority idiopathic; rarely intrinsic/extrinsic obstruction
Pulmonary sling [7]	Usually entire right lung, occasionally atelectatic right middle/lower lung	(Total) Right-sided emphysema low left hilus; anterior bowing right main bronchus	Left pulmonary artery arises from right pulmonary artery "sling" around right pulmonary artery
Massive dilatation of pulmonary artery [5a]	Usually right middle or left upper lobe	Emphysema + large hilar density	Congenital avalvular pulmonar artery [5a]; also poststenotic dilatation
Bronchogenic cyst [10][b]	usually entire right or left side	Unilateral emphysema; broad indentation of esophagus and trachea/bronchus; sometimes mediastinal mass	Bronchogenic cyst

[a] Depending on the phase, the emphysema may present radiologically in various ways (Fig. 6).
[b] Some cases present in infancy, as in the older child or adult, without respiratory impairment [10].

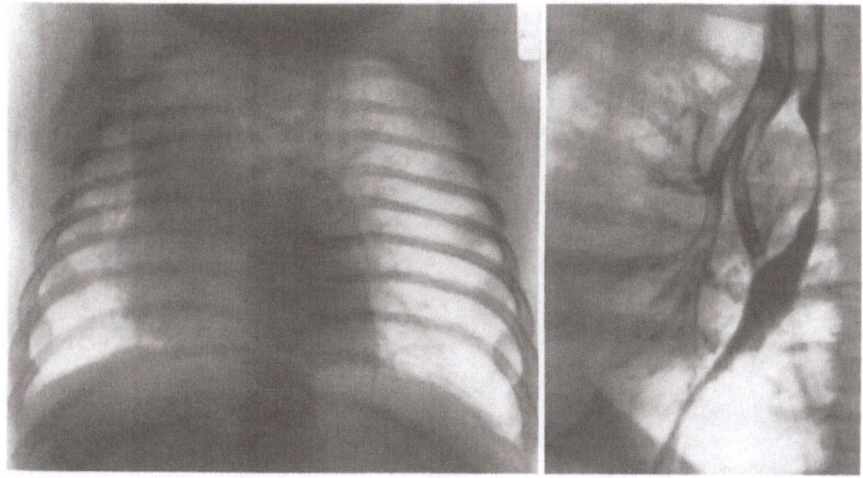

Fig. 5a and b. Female premature baby, 2 months old.
a) Unilateral hyperlucent lung (alveolar emphysema).
b) Combined tracheobronchography and esophagog-

raphy discloses bronchogenic cyst compressing mainly
left bronchus

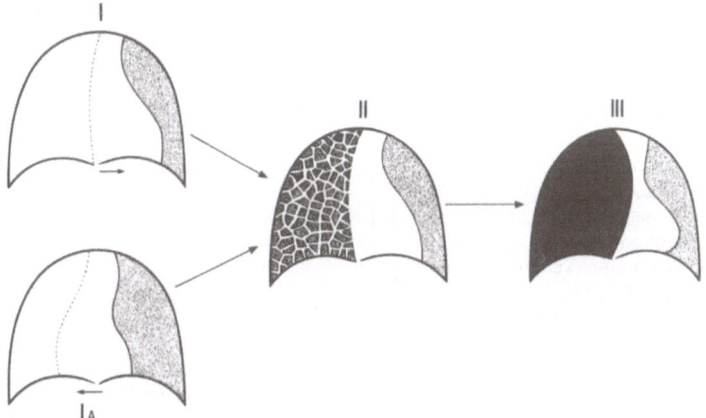

Fig. 6. Alveolar unilateral emphysema in newborn.
Schematic drawing of various phases. *I*. Retention of
intraalveolar fluid, space-occupying white mass. *I A*.
Same as *I*, but combined with some diminished vol-

ume of the affected lung. *II*. Transportation phase of
alveolar fluid through lymphatics (reticular pattern;
see Fig. 10c). *III*. Classic unilateral hyperlucent, over-
expanded lung

creasing frequency. This finding must alert the
physician to further complications (tension pneumothorax, pneumopericardium etc. (Table 6).
Again, a spectrum of four radiologic main patterns can be observed [24] (Table 5, Fig. 3, 8b–d,
h). *Isolated pulmonary lymphangiectasis* may present as a round airspace pattern (Fig. 8g). In at
least one case [14] associated hypoplasia of the
bronchial cartilage might have been a contribu-
tory factor to the airway dilatation. This pattern,

also described as reticulonodular [36], has been
seen only in primary, isolated, congenital lymphangiectasis (group III of Noonan [30]): Apparently however, some cases just show the well-
known pattern of interstitial pulmonary edema
[36].

Cystic adenomatoid malformation may show a very
similar, yet unilateral pattern: Again, this histologic diagnosis encompasses the whole spectrum
from these multicystic lesions (73.3%) (Fig. 9a), to

Table 5[*]   A. Round air space pattern

	a) Airspace $\varnothing$[a]	b) Relation wall $\varnothing$[a] to air space $\varnothing$	Remarks
Hyaline membrane p. classic reticulo granular p.	0.6–1.0 mm	> a	Dynamic changes to other stages [15]; same pattern also in pulmonary hemorrhage and early onset streptococcal infection
Interstitial miliary emphysema	circa 1 mm	$\geqq$ a	History of positive pressure breathing; other patterns: pseudo-cystic-bullous-linear
Pulmonary (isolated) lymphangiectasis	circa 2 mm	< a, Also patches	Survival only a few days or weeks
Cystic adenomatoid malformation		< a, Also patches	Unilateral
Mikity-Wilson syndrome stage I and broncho-pulmonal dysplasia stage III	1.5 mm+	< a	Perinatal history (premature/respirator)
(Diaphragmatic hernia) (cystic adenomatoid malformation)	10 mm+	< < < < a	Sunken-in abdomen, etc.

B. Reticular—"interstitial" pattern

	"Interstitial lines" $\varnothing$[a]	Remarks
1. Beginning interstitial edema	0.6 mm	
2. Alveolar fluid transport (e.g., in alveolar emphysema)	1.3 mm	Initially white lung, later black lung
3. Congenital high pressure in pulmonar veins, e.g., total anomalous venous return type III [20]	1.6 mm	Often normal heart size. May become patchy, later alveolar edema
4. Various "interstitial" pneumonias	Similar B 1	

(Spectrum)

C. Irregular Patterns

Coarse irregular pattern (fetal aspiration syndrome)	Coarse patchy irregular infiltrates, 0.5 × 0.5 mm →9 × 3 mm →confluent local and/or general overinflation	Typical spectrum. Rapid clearing in few days. Typical perinatal history
Various neonatal pneumonia patterns		Various pneumonias and pulmonary hemorrhage may display similar features

[*]   Modified from [16].
[a]   These are approximate, average figures from a few cases. They should not be considered as Scientific, accurate data, but of qualitative character.

dominant cysts in multicystic background (13.3%) and to solid homogeneous masses (13.3%) [27].
The Mikity-Wilson pattern stage I [28] (Fig. 8e) and broncho-pulmonary dysplasia stage III ("cystic appearance" [31] (Fig. 8f)) may look identical:

We have observed the latter developing as early as the 3rd day of life, obviously still in the neonatal phase.

The Reticular Interstitial-Nodular Pattern (Table 5B, Figs. 10 and 11). The pure interstitial pat-

Table 6. Clinical significance of dx interstitial pulmonary emphysema

Direct:	Stiffening of lung/space-occupying lesion
Warning sign of:	Tension pneumothorax?
	Pneumopericardium?
	Air embolism? [37]
	Potter syndrome?

tern caused by noninfectious edema and pulmonary infection may look radiologically alike (compare Figs. 10 and 11). The "fluid transportation phase" (see above) of alveolar emphysema is particularly impressive (Figs. 6, 10, c). Interstitial edema in cases of increased pulmonary venous pressure [20] may be misunderstood as infection. This holds particularly true for total anomalous pulmonary venous return below the diaphragm, type III [9], as the heart in these cases may be of normal size and cyanosis may still be absent [20] (Fig. 10 b).

The various types of regular patterns indicative of pneumonias again show the full spectrum from an early interstitial edema-like network (Fig. 11 a) to a coarse granular (Fig. 11 b) and an irregular patchy pattern (Fig. 11 e). Bomsel et al. [5] recognize a "quite typical symmetrical pattern of blurred, alveolar opacities" (nodular), the "inversion of the miliary interstitial emphysema pattern," indicative of hematogenous dissemination of streptococcal infection. In our experience, this pattern is also seen in other types of infection, e.g. listeria (Fig. 11 b), and the clinician should be alerted to secure material from stomach, rectum, lumbar fluid and blood, to come to the correct bacteriologic diagnosis.

The Irregular Pattern (Table 5 c, Fig. 11 c–e). The classical "coarse, irregular pattern" [33] (Fig. 11 d) of the fetal meconium aspiration syndrome is part

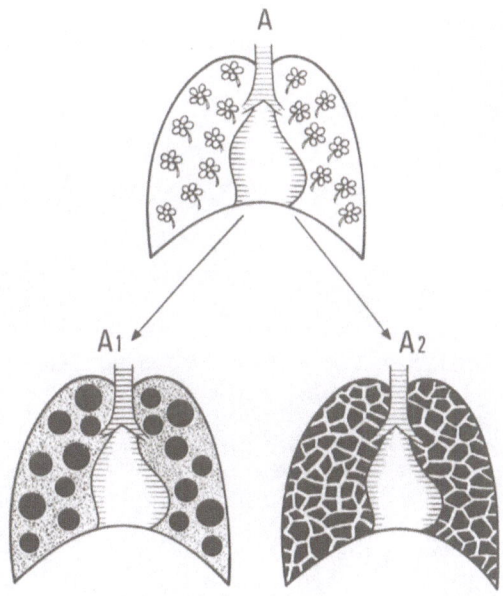

Fig. 7. Schematic drawing of "regular patterns" (A) which may be divided in round-airspace patterns (A 1) and reticular-interstitial-nodular patterns (A 2)

of a wide spectrum, ranging from minimal findings to the white chest [17].

Pneumonia, hemorrhage, and atelectasis may all contribute to a highly irregular pattern in a chest film. The correct diagnosis will depend largely on additional clinical information, as well as the radiological sequence of events with its change of patterns.

3. Conclusion

Our diagnostic approach is necessarily a static one. Quite often, the four-dimensional approach will offer valuable diagnostic hints. Finally, all enumerated and additional factors do not act in a vacuum. Sometimes, our diagnosis will, at best, be but an educated guess. Still, let's try to be radiologists first!

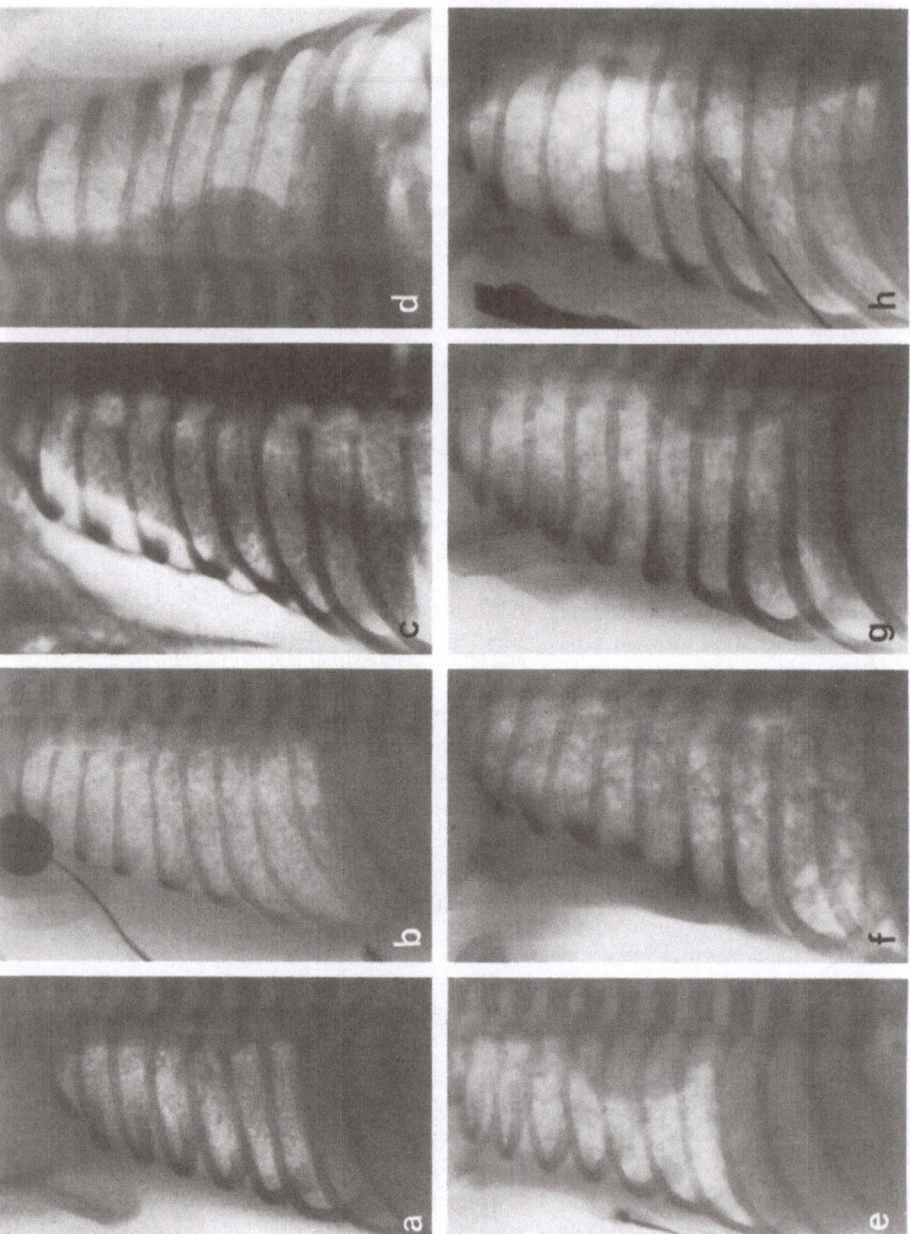

Fig. 8a–h. The round air space patterns. a) Reticulogranular pattern, hyaline membrane disease, stage I [15], 1 day old. b) Miliary interstitial emphysema, same as Fig. 3, 2 days old. c) As b), with severe *generalized* interstitial emphysema, 4 days old. d) Interstitial emphysema, *linear* type (does not belong to this group of pattern), 40 min after onset of PEEP; 3 h earlier chest radiograph normal! e) Mikity-Wilson syndrome, 7 days old. f) Bronchopulmonary dysplasia, 2 weeks old. g) Idiopathic pulmonary lymphangiectasis, 2 h old. (From [14]). h) Bullous interstitial emphysema (pneumothorax), 4 days old

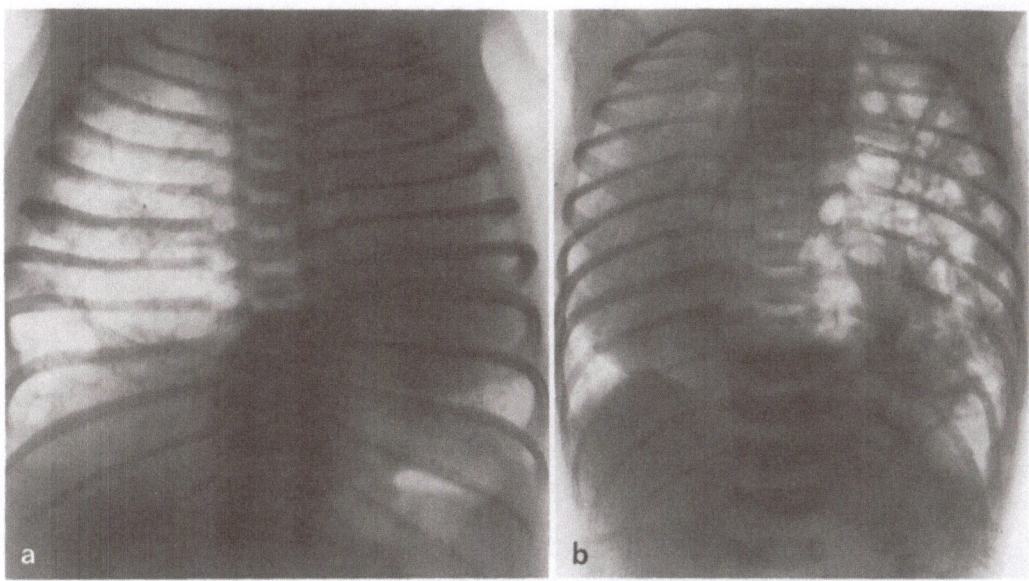

Fig. 9a and b. Round air space pattern, continued. a) Cystic adenomatoid malformation of the right lung. Multicystic type, 7 days old. b) Diaphragmatic hernia, few hours old. Notice superficial similarity of chest findings to a. Different *abdominal* air pattern

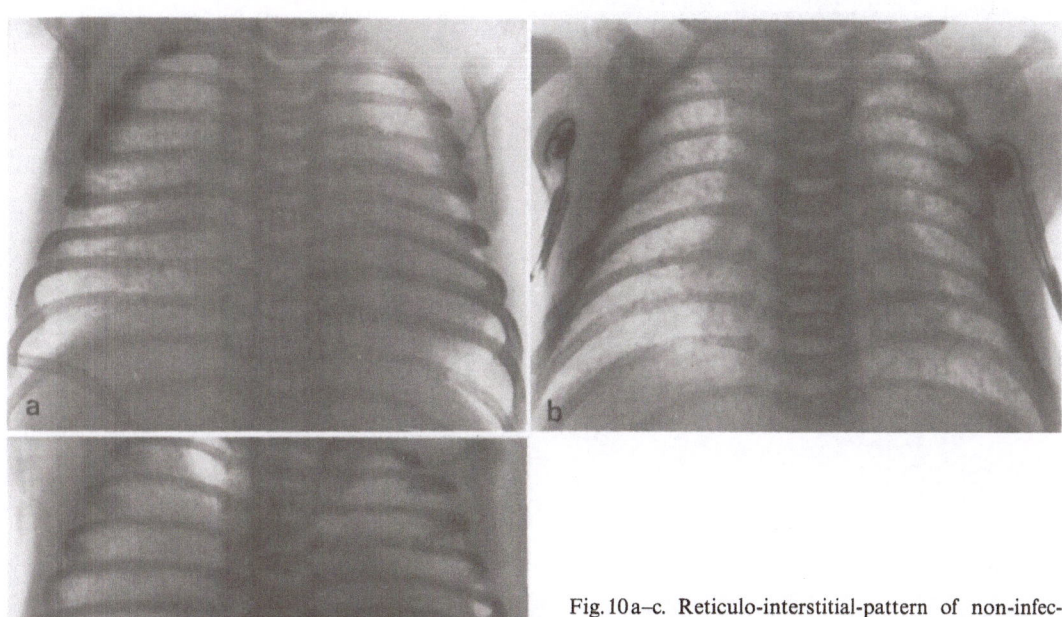

Fig. 10a–c. Reticulo-interstitial-pattern of non-infectious origin. a) Cardiac insufficiency with interstitial edema (large VSD). Enlarged heart. Female 8 days old. b) Total anomalous venous return below the diaphragm (type III [9]), male 4 days old. Notice *normal* heart size at this early age. c) Alveolar right sided emphysema, secondary to poststenotic dilatation of pulmonary artery. Displacement of mediastinal structures to the left side. (By courtesy Dr. H. Tschäppeler, Kinderspital Bern.) Male 3 h old

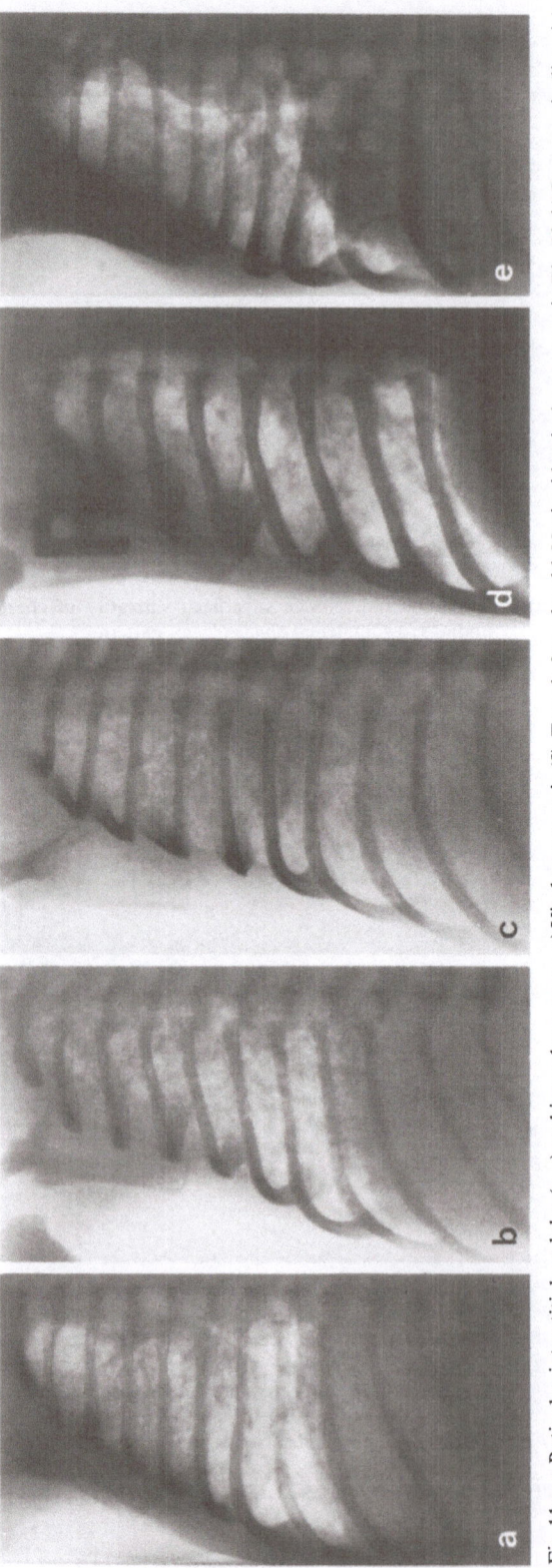

Fig. 11 a–e. Reticular-interstitial-nodular (a–c) and irregular pattern. a) Viral pneumonia (?). Female 2 weeks old. Notice identical pattern as in Fig. 10. b) Pneumonia (listeria) male 4 h old. c) Massive, non-infectious aspiration of amniotic fluid. Male 3 h. 2 days later normal chest. d) Meconium aspiration syndrome (postmaturity). Male 2 days old. e) Pneumonia (listeria). Female 4 days old

References

1. ABLOW,R.C.: Radiologic diagnosis of the newborn chest. Curr. Probl. Pediat. **1** (1971)
2. ABLOW,R.C., DRISCOLL,S.G., EFFMANN,E.L., GROSS,I., JOLLES,C.J., UAUY,R., WARSHAW,J.B.: A comparison of early onset group B streptococcal neonatal infection and the respiratorydistress syndrome of the newborn. New Engl. J. Med. **294**, 65—70 (1976)
3. ALLEN,R.P., TAYLOR,R.L., REIQUAM,C.W.: Congenital lobar emphysema with dilated septal lymphatics Radiology **86**, 929—931 (1966)
4. AVERY,M.E., FLETCHER,B.D.: The lung and its Disorders in the Newborn Infant. 3rd ed. Philadelphia: Saunders 1974
5. BOMSEL,F., COUCHARD,M., LARROCHE,J.-CL., BONAMICI,T.: Etude radiologique de l'infection pulmonaire néonatale Ann. Radiol. **19**, 87—101 (1976)
5a. BORG,S.A., YOUNG,L.W., ROGHAIR,G.D.: Congenital avalvular pulmonary artery and infantile lobar emphysema. Amer. J. Roentgenol. **125**, 412—421 (1975)
6. CAMPBELL,R.E.: Intrapulmonary interstitial emphysema: a complication of hyaline membrane disease. Amer. J. Roentgenol. **110**, 450—456 (1970)
7. CAPITANIO,M.A., RAMOS,R., KIRKPATRICK,J.A.: Pulmonary sling—roentgen observations. Amer. J. Roentgenol. **112**, 28—34 (1971)
8. CORBETT,D.P., WASHINGTON,J.E., Respiratory obstruction in the newborn and excess pulmonary fluid. Amer. J. Roentgenol. **112**, 18—22 (1971)
9. DARLING,R.C., ROTHNEY,W.B., CRAIG,J.M.: Total pulmonary venous drainage into the right side of the heart. Lab. Invest. **6**, 44—64 (1957)
10. ERAKLIS,A.J., GRISCOM,N.T., McGOVERN,J.B.: Bronchogenic Cysts of the Mediastinum in Infancy. New Engl. J. Med. **281**, 1150—1155 (1969)
11. FAWCITT,J., LIND,J., WEGELIUS,C.: The first breath. Acta paediat., Scand. (Stockholm) **49**, Suppl. 123 5—17 (1960)
11a. FRIEDLAND,G.W., AXMAN,M.M., LOVE,T.: Neonatal "urinothorax" associated with posterior urethral valves. Brit. J. Radiol. **44**, 471—474 (1971)
12. GIEDION,A.: Beidseitiger Hydrothorax als Ursache schwerster initialer Atemnot des Neugeborenen. Ein neues — nur radiologisch erfaßbares Krankheitsbild. Fortschr. Röntgenstr. **102**, 29—35 (1965)
13. GIEDION,A.: Die Atemnot des Neugeborenen in radiologischer Sicht. Pädiat. Pädol. **3**, 201—212 (1967)
14. GIEDION,A., MÜLLER,W.A., MOLZ,G.: Angeborene Lymphangiektasie der Lungen. Eine radiologisch erkennbare Ursache des Atemnotsyndroms beim Neugeborenen. Helv. Paed. Acta **22**, 170—180 (1967)

15. GIEDION,A., HAEFLIGER,H., DANGEL,P.: Acute pulmonary X-Ray changes in hyaline membrane disease treated with Artificial ventilation and positive end-expiratory pressure (PEP). Pediat. Radiol. **1**, 145—152 (1973)
16. GIEDION,A.: Radiological primer for respiratory distress in the newborn. Diagnostic Radiology 1975, 1—10. MARGULIS,A., and GOODING,C.A., eds. University of California at San Francisco 1975
17. GOODING,C.A., GREGORY,G.A.: Roentgenographic analysis of meconium aspiration of the newborn. Radiology **100**, 131—135 (1971)
18. GRISCOM,N.T., HARRIS,G.B.C., WOHL,M.E.B., VAWTER,F.G., ERAKLIS,A.J.: Fluid-filled lung due to airway obstruction in the newborn. Pediatrics **43**, 383—390 (1969)
19. GYEPES,M.T., VINCENT,W.R.: Severe Congenital Heart Disease in the Neonatal Period. Amer. J. Roentgenol. **116**, 490—500 (1972)
20. HARRIS,G.B.C., NEUHAUSER,E.B.D., GIEDION,A.: Total anomalous pulmonary venous return below the diaphragm. Amer. J. Roentgenol. **84**, 436—441 (1960)
21. HENDREN,W.H., McKEE,D.M.: Lobar emphysema of infancy. J. Pediat. Surg. **1**, 23—39 (1966)
22. KIRKPATRICK,J.A.: Roentgen diagnosis of congenital heart disease in the first months of life. Refresher course 1208. Syracuse: The Radiological Soc. North America 1973
23. KNIGHT,L., TOBIN,J., L'HEUREX,P.: Hydrothorax: A complication of hyperalimentation with radiologic manifestations. Radiology **111**, 693—695 (1974)
24. LALLEMAND,D., TRAN VAN DUC, SAUVEGRAIN,J.: When does interstitial emphysema become visible? Ann. Radiol. **16**, 58—61 (1973)
25. LOHER,E., GIEDION,A.: Radiological aspects of massive pulmonary hemorrhage in the newvorn. Ann. Radiol. **14**, 147—154 (1971)
26. MacEVAN,D.W., DUNBAR,J.S., SMITH,R.D., BROWN,B.ST.J.: Pneumothorax in the neonate (its recognition and evaluation). Ann. Radiol. **7**, 459 (1964)
27. MADEWELL, J.E., STOCKER,T., KORSOWER,J.M.: Cystic adenomatoid malformation of the lung. Amer. J. Roentgenol. **124**, 436—448 (1975)
28. MIKITY,V.G., HODGMAN,J.E., TATTER,D.: The radiological findings in delayed pulmonary maturation in premature infants. Progr. Pediat. Radiol. **1**, 149—159 (1976)
29. NADELHAFT,J., ELLIS,K.: Roentgen appearance of the lungs in 1000 apparently normal full term newborn infants. Amer. J. Roentgenol. **78**, 440—443 (1957)
30. NOONAN,J.A., WALTERS,L.R., REEVES,J.T.: Congenital pulmonary lymphangiectasis. Amer. J. Dis. Child. **120**, 314—319 (1970)

31. NORTHWAY, W. H., ROSAN, R. C.: Radiographic features of pulmonary oxygen toxicity in the newborn: Bronchopulmonary dysplasia. Radiology 91, 49—58 (1968)

32. OESTREICH, A.: The sharp edge sign in neonatal pneumothorax. Paper read at the ESPR congress May 1976, Stockholm

33. PETERSON, H. G., PENDLETON, M. E.: Contrasting roentgenographic pulmonary patterns of the hyaline membrane and fetal aspiration syndromes. Amer. J. Roentgenol. 74, 800—813 (1955)

34. Symposium on neonatal radiology. REILLY, B. J. (Ed.) Radiol. clin. North America 13, No. 2 (1975)

35. SEIBERT, J. J., WEINSTEIN, M. M., ERENBERG, A.: Catheter-related complications of total parenteral nutrition in infants. Pediat. Radiol. 4, 233—237 (1976)

36. SHANNON, M. P., GRANTMYRE, E. B., REID, W. D., WOTHERSPOON, A. S.: Congenital pulmonary lymphangiectasis. Pediat. Radiol. 2, 235—240 (1974)

37. SIEGLE, R. L., EYAL, F. G., RABINOWITZ, J. G.: Air embolus following pulmonary interstitial emphysema in hyaline membrane disease. Clin. Radiol. 27, 77—80 (1976)

38. SWISCHUK, L. E.: Radiology of the Newborn and Young Infant. Baltimore: Williams and Williams 1973

38a. VOLLMAN, J. H., SMITH, W. L., BALLARD, E. T., LIGHT, I. J.: Early onset group B streptococcal disease—clinical, roentgenographic, and pathologic features. J. Pediat. 89, 199—204 (1976)

39. WEIGEL, W., MENTZEL, H.: Die angeborene Lymphangiektasie der Lunge. Mschr. Kinderheilk. 122, 85—87 (1974)

40. WELLER, M. H., KATZENSTEIN, A. A.: Radiological finding in group B streptococcal sepsis. Radiology 118, 385—387 (1976)

41. WESENBERG, R. L.: The Newborn Chest. Hagerstown, Md., Harper, and Row 1973

Chronic Lung Disorders in Childhood

F. N. Silverman

1. Indroduction

A review of chronic lung disorders in childhood might be developed on the basis of conditions present in premature infants, term infants, toddlers, etc; but some disorders occur in all age groups. An alternative would be to base the review on radiographic patterns; but many conditions have similar patterns, and specificity with respect to cause is poor. However, the combination of pattern *and* age can provide clues to etiology, and consequently can contribute to treatment.

In general, chronic lung disorders include conditions characterized *clinically* by respiratory symptoms or signs of weeks' to months' duration, and *radiologically* by diffuse, patchy areas of increased density and/or radiolucency, frequently with prominent hilar components. Additional signs of chronic disease may be present in extrarespiratory system sites; transverse, post growth-arrest lines in metaphyseal areas, osteoporosis, paucity of subcutaneous fat and other fat depots, etc. Segmental or lobar involvement may occur, but these are more frequent in acute diseases.

2. Chronic Aspiration Pneumonia

Chronic aspiration may be a manifestation of various primary disorders. Anatomical malformations such as tracheo-esophageal fistulas, with and without congenital atresia of the esophagus and its variants, can be mimicked by pathophysiologic disorders in which there is delay or even failure of development of some of the basal nuclei required for maintaining a normal swallowing mechanism (Fig. 1). Material aspirated into the trachea, responding to the increased size and more direct continuation of the right maintends bronchus than the left, tends to lodge in bronchial divisions arising from the right side. In the recumbent infant, the right upper lobe is frequently involved; the bases of both lungs are not infrequently affected. The foreign material, either by itself or by the inflammatory reaction that results, produces varying degrees of obstruction which can give rise to irregular emphysema, irregular atelectasis with linear streaks radiating out from the hilum, and secondary inflammatory reaction. The radiating streaks going out from the hila probably represent segmental collapse of portions of lung with major dimensions parallel to the beam of X-rays passing through the chest. When segments of collapse (and/or inflammatory reaction) are transversed

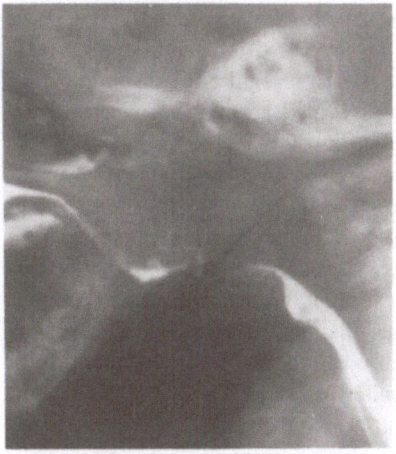

Fig. 1. Disordered swallowing mechanism indicated by reflux of contrast agent into the nasopharynx. Probably delayed maturation of control (basal ganglia?) as child had spontaneous clinical recovery after 9 months of age

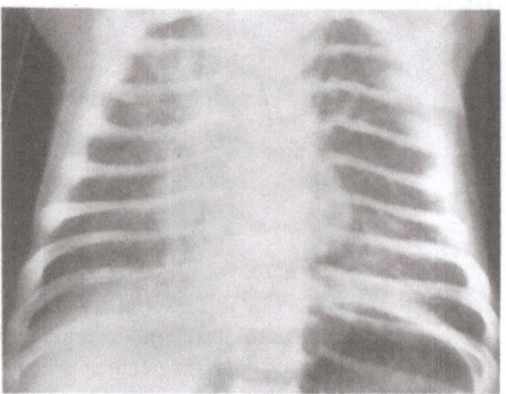

Fig. 2. Chronic and recurrent aspiration pneumonia in a 9-month infant with "H" type tracheo-esophageal fistula

obliquely or *en face*, they may contribute only to the ill-defined increased density in the area of involvement. To study properly the relationship between esophagus and trachea, examination of the swallowing mechanism in physiologic deglutition may have to be supplemented by mechanical distention of the esophagus via a nasogastric tube. Recurrent aspiration often follows surgical correction of a congenital atresia of the esophagus with or without a fistula, or a fistula with or without atresia (Fig. 2). In such instances, contrast demonstration of a fistulous communication may represent recurrence of a fistula, but may also be an indication of pre-existing additional fistulas which had not been recognized initially. The difficulty of passage of a peristaltic wave from the upper segment into the lower segment may also be responsible for recurrent aspiration. The relatively narrow site of anastomosis seldom represents a real stricture, and the pathophysiologic disturbance is probably an associated abnormality of innervation of the two segments of the esophagus rather than a consequence of the surgical intervention. When the features of fistula are present, but swallowing difficulties and fistula formation are not clearly recognized, the rare occurrence of posterior laryngeal clefts has to be considered.

Recently, attention has been drawn to many other types of abnormal respiratory/alimentary communications which can be associated with chronic pneumonia. A bronchus may arise directly from the esophagus, or communications may exist with the gastrointestinal system below the diaphragm. An instance of biliary-bronchial fistula has been reported, in which the production of greenish sputum provided the indication for a contrast examination which demonstrated the fistulous communication. When considering aspiration pneumonia, one should not overlook the chronic inflammatory reactions that result from foreign bodies, such as grass, pine, needles, broomstraws, etc., which of themselves are radiolucent but which can persist and produce severe recurrent disease. The tendency for such conditions to remain fairly sharply localized, in spite of spread to other portions of the lung in different episodes, indicates the area to be examined most carefully endoscopically and/or in association with contrast agents. Children with recurrent regurgitation but no true obstruction may also aspirate. Recognition of chalasia and/or hiatus hernia and their treatment can lead to cure.

Defective swallowing mechanisms and esophageal motility as a manifestation of familial dysautonomia (Riley-Day syndrome) probably contribute to the frequent pneumonia seen in children with this condition. Other evidence of neuromuscular incoordination, including scoliosis, in association with chronic or recurring pneumonia, warrants consideration of this condition. Brain damage of various types may be associated with swallowing difficulties and aspiration.

3. Congenital Malformations

Apart from the contributions to chronic aspiration, congenital malformations of the respiratory tract may be associated with chronic lung disease on other bases. Aplasia or hypoplasia of a lung may simulate chronic disease because of the aeration disturbance found in the course of an acute superimposed infection (Fig. 3). Careful correlation with the clinical signs of chronic and/or recurrent pulmonary disease is important in order to avoid unnecessary manipulative procedures. Persistent and/or progressively worsening respiratory symptoms may require intervention. In the

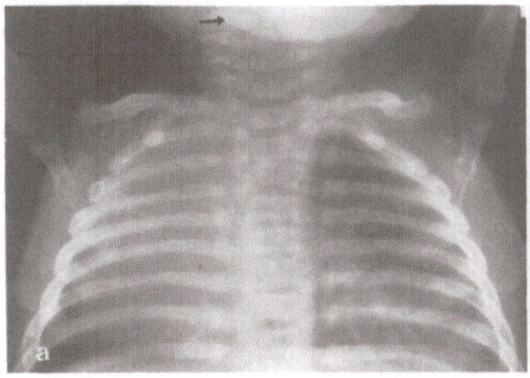

Fig. 3a and b. Pulmonary hypoplasia (actually, aplasia of right lung) masquerading as chronic respiratory disease. Abnormal radiograph persisting after clinical recovery from acute respiratory infection was considered as manifestation of chronic, acquired disease

a) Cervical hemivertrebra in tele-roentgenogram was thought to indicate possible malformation basis for findings
b) Bronchogram demonstrated absence of right bronchial tree and lung, with herniation of left lower lobe into right hemithorax

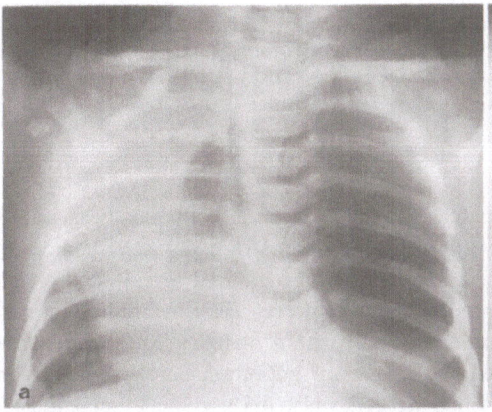
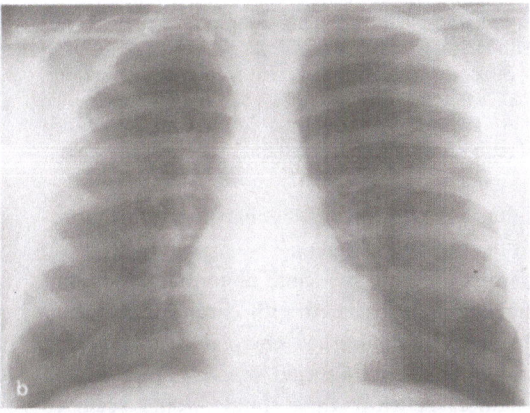

Fig. 4a and b. Congenital lobar emphysema and its evolution
a) Age, 3 months. Persistent respiratory distress since birth; family refused surgical intervention despite episodes of severe cyanosis

b) Age, 9 years. Shortness of breath on exertion only; otherwise, normally developed. Note relative increase in size of left hemithorax compared to right, and diminished vascular markings and increased radiolucency of left upper hemithorax. Is this one mechanism of the Swyer-James syndrome?

newborn, lobar emphysema is generally not considered a cause of chronic disease; however, if unrecognized, or if surgical treatment is not undertaken, it may contribute to the incidence of chronic disease in later life (Fig. 4). Likewise, cystic disease of lung, usually presenting as cystic adenomatoid malformation of the lung, may be a cause of later morbidity. Sequestration of the lung, frequently requiring angiographic procedures for diagnosis, commonly presents with recurring respi-

ratory symptoms. The lack of communication with the remainder of the tracheobronchial tree, which prevents the drainage of infected material, probably plays a role in perpetuating infection in the sequestered pulmonary tissue. I have encountered an unexpected instance of congenital sequestration of the lung in a patient who otherwise clinically had the features of Kartagener's syndrome (Fig. 5). The possibility that this form of malformation contributes to the pulmonary man-

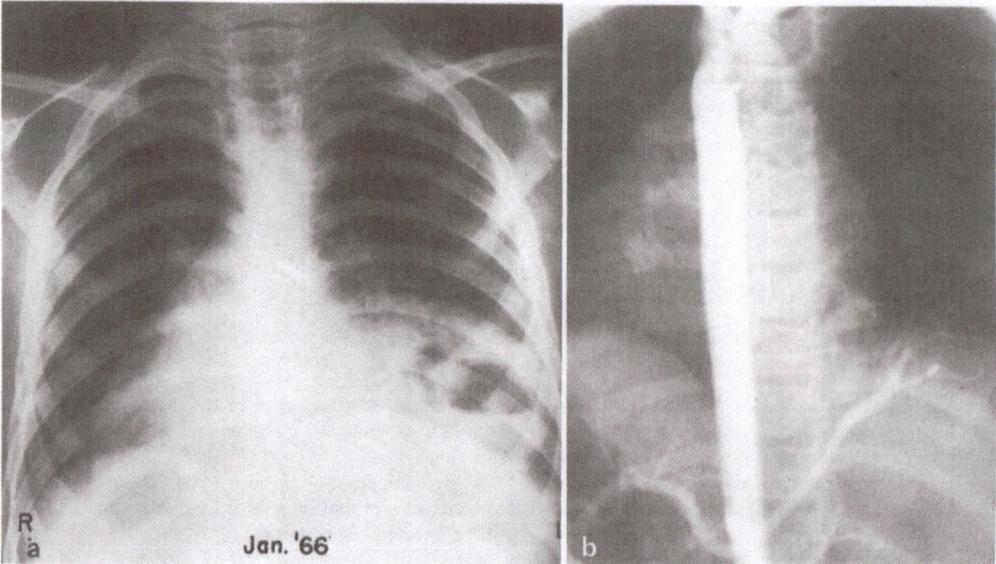

Fig. 5a and b. Chronic lung disease in 8-year-old girl with the diagnosis of Kartagener syndrome on basis of a) Situs inversus, with recurrent respiratory infections, and "cystic bronchiectasis". When it was appreciated that patient had no sputum or foul breath, a diagnosis of sequestration was suggested

b) Aortogram demonstrated anomalous arterial supply. Extralobar sequestration removed surgically with complete cure of respiratory symptoms

ifestations of the syndrome may merit further investigation.

Cardiac and cardiovascular abnormalities are not infrequently associated with chronic respiratory disease. The diminished compliance of the lung due to splinting by turgid vascular structures in instances of left-to-right shunts would seem to limit the lung's capability to overcome infection; pressure by enlarged vessels or abnormal vessels, such as in the case of vascular rings, may also interfere with normal aeration, and perhaps drainage of the lungs.

4. Allergic Diseases

Allergic diseases in childhood, exemplified by asthma, may be a cause of considerable morbidity and even mortality. Radiographically, the pattern of severe generalized emphysema with some prominence of the bronchovascular markings after recurrent attacks permits the diagnosis. The patchy pneumonias, seen so frequently in adults with recurrent asthma, are not so common in children in whom generalized severe emphysema predominates. However, persistent radiologic disease can occur with a changing pattern in which emphysema is an important constituent, but in which there may also develop small foci of atelectasis and/or pneumonia. It is important to recognize that a foreign body that changes its position within the respiratory tract can produce similar clinical and radiographic manifestations.

Some children appear to be allergic to milk (presumably milk proteins) and may have recurrent respiratory signs and symptoms as a consequence. The relation of the clinical and radiologic manifestations to the exposure to or withdrawal of milk products may be used to support this somewhat uncertain diagnosis (Fig. 6). The historical aspects of exposure to respiratory allergens may also explain chronic and/or recurrent respiratory changes in children who have hypersensitivity to birds, animals, and various forms of air pollutants. Recent reports of recurrent respiratory disease, secondary to exposure to spores of certain

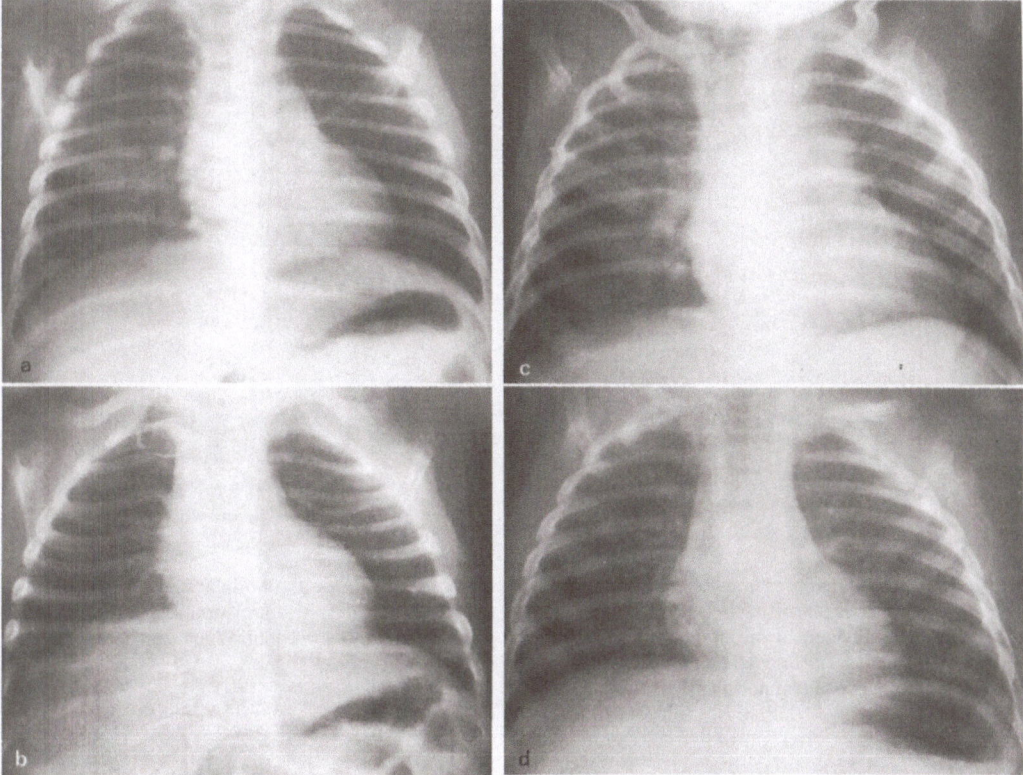

Fig. 6 a–d. Probable example of pulmonary response in allergy to milk. Male, $3\frac{1}{2}$ months old. Respiratory symptoms noted after beginning of artificial feeding (cow's milk) at 6 weeks
a) Feb. 12, admission film; diffuse consolidation in right mid hemithorax

b) Feb. 16, after 4 days on diet without cow's milk
c) Mar. 20, after deliberate reintroduction of cow's milk. Patchy densities recur together with clinical signs of cough, rales, and some wheezing
d) Mar. 25, after removing milk from diet

forms of thermophilic fungi which have contaminated filters in air conditioning units have provided another source for investigation when recurrent pulmonary infection is noted.

5. Systemic Diseases

One of the best-known causes of chronic lung disease in childhood is mucoviscidosis or cystic fibrosis of the pancreas. The radiographic hallmarks of the disease—pulmonary hyperaeration, increased bronchovascular markings with peribronchial cuffing, hilar adenomegaly, and disseminated patchy consolidations (Fig. 7)—have their origin in the abnormal secretions and abnormal ciliary activity in the lungs of affected individuals. The patchy densities which leave cystic bronchiectatic changes when they disappear are now recognized as manifestations of thick mucoid impactions in the dilated bronchi. Radiographic features, including bronchial concretions simulating mucous plugs, have been described in pulmonary infection with Bordetella bronchiseptica. Other features of cystic fibrosis can be recognized radiographically in the respiratory tract and include nasal fibromas and polyps. We have observed one instance in which a mucous retention cyst in an ethmoid sinus, simulating a malignant neoplasm, led to the diagnosis of the systemic disease. Radiographic features in the gastrointestinal tract are

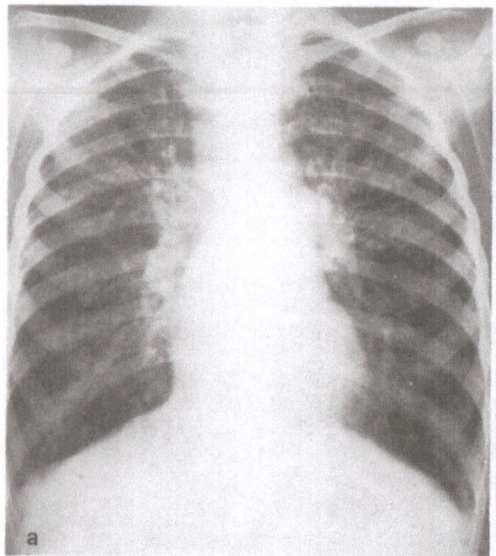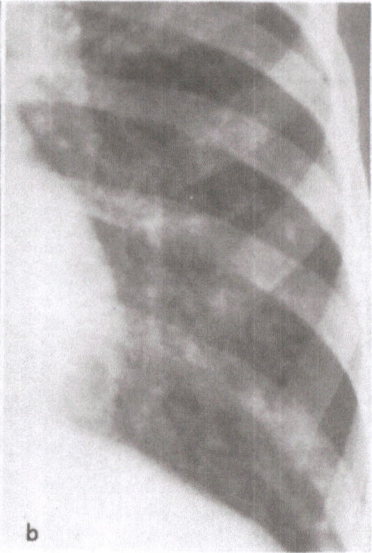

Fig. 7a and b. Pulmonary features of cystic fibrosis of the pancreas (mucoviscidosis)
a) 3-year female. Prominent hilum (adenopathy), "honeycombing", and peribronchial "cuffing", hyperaeration and multiple peripheral nodular densities

b) Close up of linear and nodular densities in left lower lung. Nodular densities are produced by mucous impactions in dilated bronchi. When expelled, they leave radiolucent cystic changes

well known and do not concern us at this time. Atypical consolidations and clinical disease may be the result of contamination of apparatus used for respiratory therapy with unusual organisms such as *Pseudomonas aeruginosa*. This iatrogenic complication should be considered when clinical disease fails to respond to previously effective management, and when parenchymal densities are more prominent than usual for a given patient.

Disturbances of immune mechanisms may also manifest themselves by recurrent pulmonary infections. The diagnosis of agammaglobulinemia or hypogammaglobulinemia may be advanced by noting deficient adenoid tissue in a lateral film of the neck and head (Fig. 8); alternatively, excessive overgrowth of adenoid tissue may indicate hyperplasia of the structures in dysgammaglobulinemia. Absence of the usually well-developed thymus of infancy in a lateral film of a very young infant who has not been ill long enough for stress atrophy of the thymus may point toward the DiGeorge syndrome, thymic alymphoplasia. In addition, the observation of the diffuse increase in

density that accompanies infection with *Pneumocystis carinii* may point toward some disturbance in the immune mechanisms. Infection with this organism and other types of opportunistic infections are important problems in children rendered immunologically incompetent by neoplasms and/or their treatment.

In Letterer-Siwe's disease (Fig. 9), proliferation of reticuloendothelial cells in the structural framework of the lungs may produce streaky densities and emphysema not unlike those seen in association with cystic fibrosis of the pancreas. The complication of spontaneous pneumothorax must be kept in mind in both conditions. Pulmonary hemosiderosis occasionally occurs in children and may have no diagnostic radiographic features; a recurring pattern, however, is often found and the diagnosis is made by the identification of siderocytes in tracheobronchial or gastric aspirates. Some instances have been desribed as a complication of milk allergy, with disappearance of signs and symptoms when the offending product has been removed from the diet (see Fig. 6). The Hamman-Rich syndrome (Fig. 10), chronic interstitial

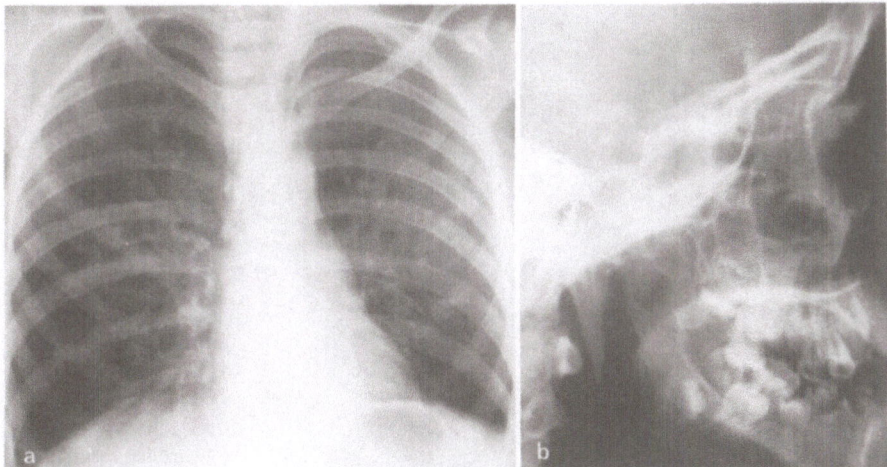

Fig. 8a and b. Hypogammaglobulinemia with recurrent respiratory infections

a) Chest at 14 years. Diffuse fibrotic and inflammatory changes
b) Nasopharynx almost devoid of adenoid tissue

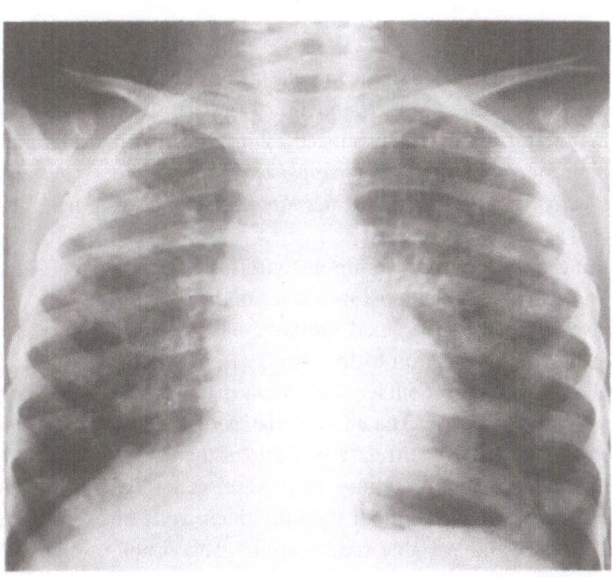

Fig. 9. Letterer-Siwe disease (Histiocytosis-X) in a 4½-year-old boy. Presented with extensive "cradle cap" and hepato-splenomegaly. Never developed any bone lesions

pulmonary fibrosis, is probably an end result of many chronic inflammatory diseases of the lung and not an entity in its own right. The radiographic features are comparable to those of any chronic pulmonary disease; increased irregular densities, areas of pulmonary over- and under-aeration, and frequently the cardiac manifestations of pulmonary hypertension. "Honeycombing" is a common radiographic feature in severe cases.

6. Chronic Infections

Certain infections have a tendency to chronicity in the lungs regardless of the immune status of the patient. These should not be overlooked in children who have pulmonary manifestations of chronic respiratory disease. In developing countries, in particular, the role of tuberculosis as a cause of chronic pulmonary morbidity cannot be

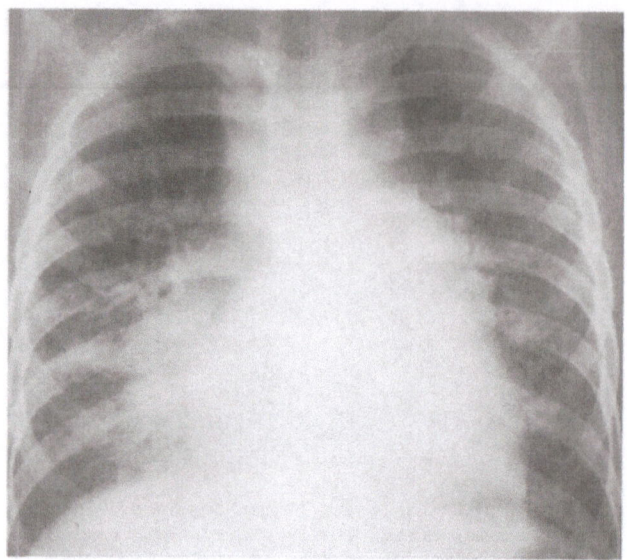

Fig. 10. Hamman-Rich syndrome in a $14^1/_2$-year-old-boy. History of chronic recurring respiratory infections with progressive respiratory failure. At this time, patient had severe pulmonary hypertension. Note "honeycombing"

forgotten. Its radiographic manifestations are well known; in other countries, identical radiographic manifestations can be produced by infection with biphasic fungi such as *Histoplasma capsulatum*, *Blastomyces dermatitidis*, *Coccidioides immitis*, as well as other organisms.

Lung abscess is an uncommon condition in childhood. Probably the most frequent condition confused with it is loculated emphysema, a consequence of obstruction to the egress of air usually occurring in the course of *recovery* from acute respiratory disease. The characteristics of the latter include lack of correlation of size of the cavity with clinical manifestations of disease, generally relatively thin walls rather than the thick walls of abscesses, and variable radiographic progression and regression without associated clinical manifestations. Fluid may often appear within these loculated "cystic" cavities within the lung. Mention is made of the condition here in order to avoid unnecessary concern over a condition such as putrid lung abscess or the probably non-existent aputrid lung abscess, and the implications with respect to surgical management which relate to true lung abscesses.

An increasing number of infants and children who present with chronic respiratory complaints, and widespread radiographic changes, are graduates of premature intensive care units; their prognosis is still uncertain but they must be considered as belonging to the children who are the subject of this survey. A history of prematurity may be very helpful in understanding the nature of chronic pulmonary disease in some instances when other considerations are not supported.

7. Conclusion

I was tempted to use a single radiograph to illustrate this review of chronic lung disorders because many of the various conditions noted above present almost identical radiologic manifestations. A diagnosis of chronic pulmonary disease in children is made on the basis of the radiologic features in the lungs, associated radiologic features elsewhere in the body, the clinical history and laboratory data. It is hoped that this review can present an abbreviated spectrum of the conditions which must come up for consideration when a child presents with clinical and radiologic signs of chronic pulmonary disease. A more complete listing of conditions than those which have been discussed is presented in Table 1.

Table 1. A listing of causes of chronic pulmonary disease in childhood

A. *Aspiration*	3. Defective defense mechanisms

A. *Aspiration*
1. Brain
a) Malformation
b) Trauma
c) Dysfunction—(Riley-Day)
2. Respiratory and Foregut
a) Laryngeal
b) Esophageal atresia
c) Tracheo-esophageal fistula
d) Vascular ring
e) Chalasia-hiatal hernia

B. *Congenital anomaly*
1. Aplasia
2. Hypoplasia
a) Anomalies of vascular supply and drainage
b) "Duplication" diaphragm
3. Lobar emphysema
4. Anomalous origin/course of left pulmonary artery
5. Cystic disease
a) Adenomatoid malformation
b) Tracheobronchial cyst (foregut cyst)
6. Sequestration
7. Duplication
8. Dysmaturity (?)
9. Kartagener syndrome

C. *Allergy*
1. Asthma
2. Loeffler
3. Milk, etc.
4. Bacterial, mycobacterial, fungal antigens

D. *Systemic disease*
1. Cystic fibrosis, pancreas
2. Riley-Day syndrome

3. Defective defense mechanisms
a) Immune globulin disturbances
b) Ataxia — telangiectasia
c) Neutropenia
d) Other cellular deficiencies
e) Wiskott-Aldrich syndrome
f) Ex-premature

E. *Physical agents*
1. Foreign bodies (nose to alveoli)
2. Hydrocarbon aspiration
3. Lipid
4. Radiation
5. Noxious gases

F. *Neoplastic*
1. Histiocytosis-X
2. Leukemia

G. *Infection*
1. Tuberculosis
2. Fungus (histoplasmosis and other bi-phasic fungi)
3. Mycoplasma
4. Viruses
5. Suppurative
6. Slowly resolving (e.g., pertussis)
7. Pneumocystis carinii
8. Giant cell pneumonia (measles)
9. Bronchiectasis

H. *Miscellaneous*
1. Sarcoid
2. Hemosiderosis
3. Alveolar proteinosis
4. Hamman-Rich
5. Other

References

1. BAKER, D. H., PARMER, E. A., WOLFF, J. A.: Roentgen manifestations of the Aldrich syndrome. Amer. J. Roentgenol. **88**, 458 (1962)
2. BANASZAK, E. F., THIEDE, W. H., FINK, J. N.: Hypersensitivity pneumonitis due to contamination of an air conditioner. N. Eng. J. Med. **283**, 277 (1970)
3. DE PARÉDÈS, C. G. et al.: Pulmonary sequestration in infants and children: a 20 years' experience and review of the literature. J. Pediat. Surg. **5**, 136 (1970)
4. DINER, W. C., KINCKER, W. T., HEINER, D. C.: Roentgenographic manifestations in the lungs in milk allergy. Radiology **77**, 564 (1961)
5. FRANK, M. M., GATEWOOD, O. M. B.: Transient pharyngeal incoordination in the newborn. Amer. J. Dis. Child. **11**, 178 (1966)
6. GEIGER, J. P. et al.: Laryngo-tracheal-esophageal cleft. J. Thoracic and Cardiovas. Surg. **59**, 330 (1970)
7. GERBEAUX, J., COUVREUR, J., TOURNIER, G.: Pathologie Respiratoire de l'Enfant. Paris: Flammarion Médicine-Sciences, 1975
8. GRISCOM, N. T.: Persistent esophagotrachea: The most persistent degree of laryngo tracheo-esophageal cleft. Amer. J. Roentgenol. **97**, 211 (1966).
9. GYEPES, M. T. et al.: Familial dysautonomia: The mechanism of aspiration. Radiology **91**, 471 (1968)
10. HEERSMA, J. A. et al.: Farmer's lung in a 10-year-old girl. J. Pediat. **75**, 704 (1969)
11. JOFFE, N.: Roentgenographic aspects of primary pseudomonas aeruginosa pneumonia in mechanically ventilated patients. Amer. J. Roentgenol. **107**, 305 (1969)
12. KIRKPATRICK, J. A. et al.: The motor activity of the esophagus in association with esophageal atresia and tracheo-esophageal fistula. Amer. J. Roentgenol. **86**, 884 (1961)
13. KIRKPATRICK, J. A.: The problem of chronic and recurrent pulmonary disease. Prog. Ped. Radiol. KAUFMANN, H. J. (ed.) **1**, 294 (1967)

14. KIRKPATRICK, J. A. et al.: Immunologic abnormalities: roentgen observations. Radiol. Clin. North Amer. **10**, 245 (1972)

15. KREPLER, P., FLAMM, H.: Bordatella bronchi-septica als Erreger menschlicher Erkrankungen. Wiener klinische Wochenschrift **70**, 641 (1958)

16. NEUHAUSER, E. B. D. et al.: Congenital direct communication between the biliary system and the respiratory tract. Amer. J. Dis. Child. **83**, 654 (1952)

17. ROGHAIR, G. D.: Non-operative management of lobar emphysema: Long-term follow-up. Radiology **102**, 125 (1972)

18. SCHWARTZ, E. E., HOLSCLAW, D. S.: Pulmonary involvement in adults with cystic fibrosis. Amer. J. Roentgenol. **122**, 708 (1974)

19. SIMON, G. et al.: Radiologic abnormalities in children with asthma and their relation to clinical findings and some respiratory function tests. Thorax **28**, 115 (1973)

20. STRAUSS, R. G., WEST, P. J., SILVERMAN, F. N.: Unilateral proptosis in cystic fibrosis. Pediatrics **43**, 297 (1969)

21. SWAYE, P. et al.: Familial Hamman Rich syndrome: report of 8 cases. Dis. Chest. **55**, 7 (1969)

22. UNGER, J. DE B., FINK, J. N., UNGER, G. F.: Pigeon breeder's disease: a review of the roentgenographic pulmonary findings. Radiology **90**, 683 (1968)

23. VANHOUTTE, J. J., GATEWOOD, O. M. B., TALBERT, J. L., BROOKER, A., HALLER, J. A. JR.: Cinefluorographic and manometric evaluation of the motor function of the esophagus following segmental resection in newborn dogs. Radiology **86**, 718 (1966)

Therapeutic Embolization of Arteriovenous Pulmonary Fistulas by Catheter Technique

W. Porstmann

1. Introduction

Arteriovenous (a–v) fistulas of the lung are abnormal communications between pulmonary arterial and venous systems. As a result, the capillary system, which ordinarily provides for gaseous exchange, is bypassed and so unoxygenated blood from the pulmonary circulation flows into the systemic circulation. A right-to-left shunt is created and the systemic arterial blood is not fully saturated with oxygen. Such fistulas are rare and are usually congenital anomalies. However, there are also acquired a–v fistulas caused by chronic inflammatory processes which are often mycotic. The fistulas may occur singly or they may be multiple in both lungs. They are frequently found with telangiectasia of the systemic circulation, as in Osler's disease.

The pathologic-anatomical finding is an angiomatous convolution or a direct arterio-venous aneurysm between a pulmonary artery and a vein. The clinical picture is determined by the size of the right-to-left shunt. In severe *pronounced* cases there is cyanosis, polycythemia, clubbing of the fingers and increased cardiac output of both the right and left ventricles. On auscultation, systolic-diastolic or continuous murmurs may be heard over the fistulas, but some fistulas are silent. A roentgenogram of the thorax shows a variable opacity, the form of which is determined by the type of fistula (angioma or aneurysm). Large vascular markings, corresponding to the afferent artery and efferent vein, suggest the presence of a fistula. This finding is especially well seen in *the* tomograms. Smaller fistulas may not be visualised on plain films of the thorax. Pulmonary angiography demonstrates the extent of the fistula and whether it is of angiomatous or aneurysmal nature. The sites (often multiple) of arterial inflow and the premature venous outflow are shown. With selective injection of contrast medium a

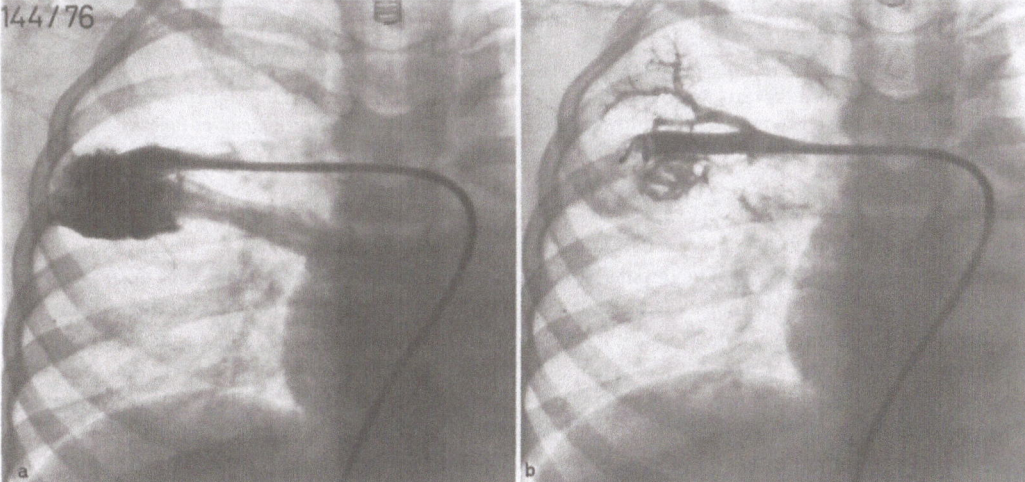

Fig. 1a and b. Angiomatous a–v pulmonary fistula in a four-year-old boy before and after embolization with a Gianturco spiral in the artery leading to the fistula

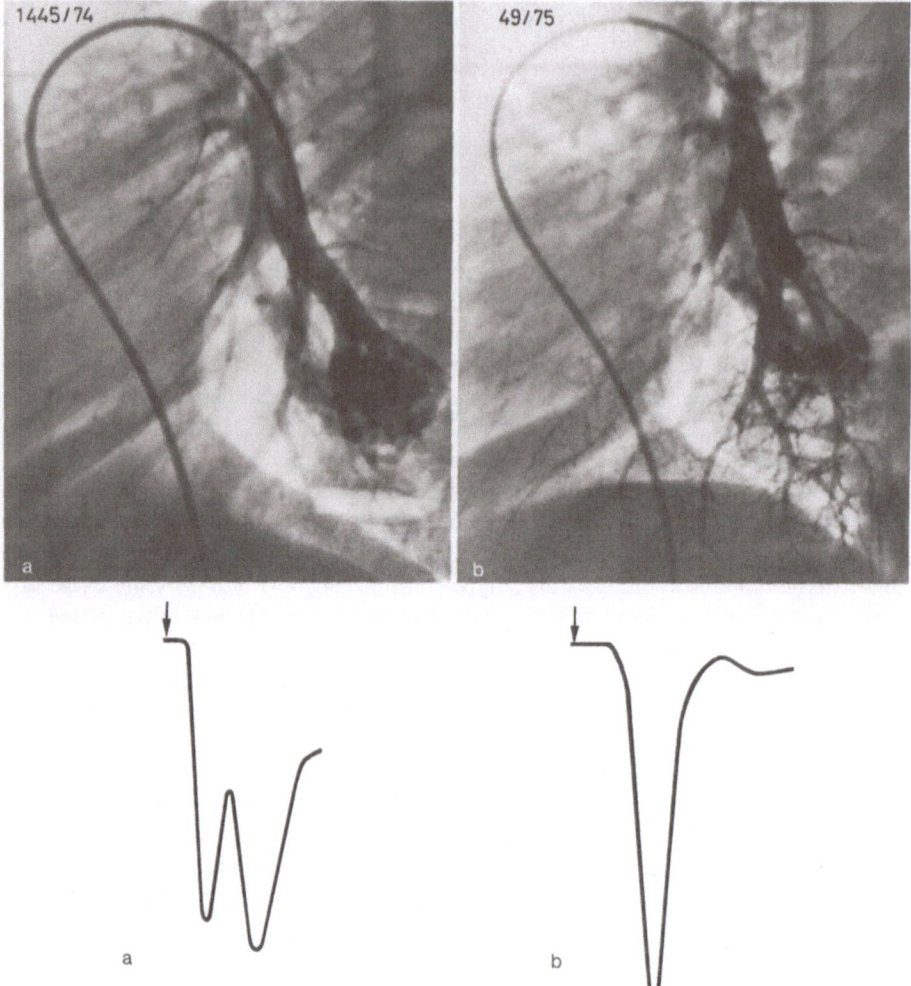

Fig. 2 and b. Clinical course of a partially closed large a–v pulmonary fistula in a 14-year-old boy
a) Angiomatous fistula in the posterobasal lower lobe segment before treatment

b) Clearly reduced size of angioma following percutaneous insertion of 20 Ivalon chips
Bottom now: Dye dilution curves (inferin vena cava—femoral artery)

characteristic of all a–v fistulas is especially well seen and this is the "steal" effect of the fistula from the normal pulmonary arteries. The detailed anatomy of the fistula *is* best demonstrated by injecting contrast medium into the afferent artery.

The treatment of a–v pulmonary fistulas is usually surgical. In most cases a lobectomy is called for. When both lungs are affected by multifocal fistulas resection is doubtful or even out of the question. Recurrences after operation are not rare.

In our experience a–v fistula may also be treated without thoracotomy by percutaneous catheteri-

zation. The goal of treatment is to block the artery leading to the fistula, and yet to take care not to damage the normal branches that do not lead to the fistula. To reach this objective the afferent pulmonary artery (usually the segmental branch) must be selectively catheterised. The material used to block the artery is then introduced through the catheter (either by injection or implantation). The procedure is controlled by injecting contrast medium through the therapeutic catheter and monitoring progress by video tape, cineradiography or serial angiographic record-

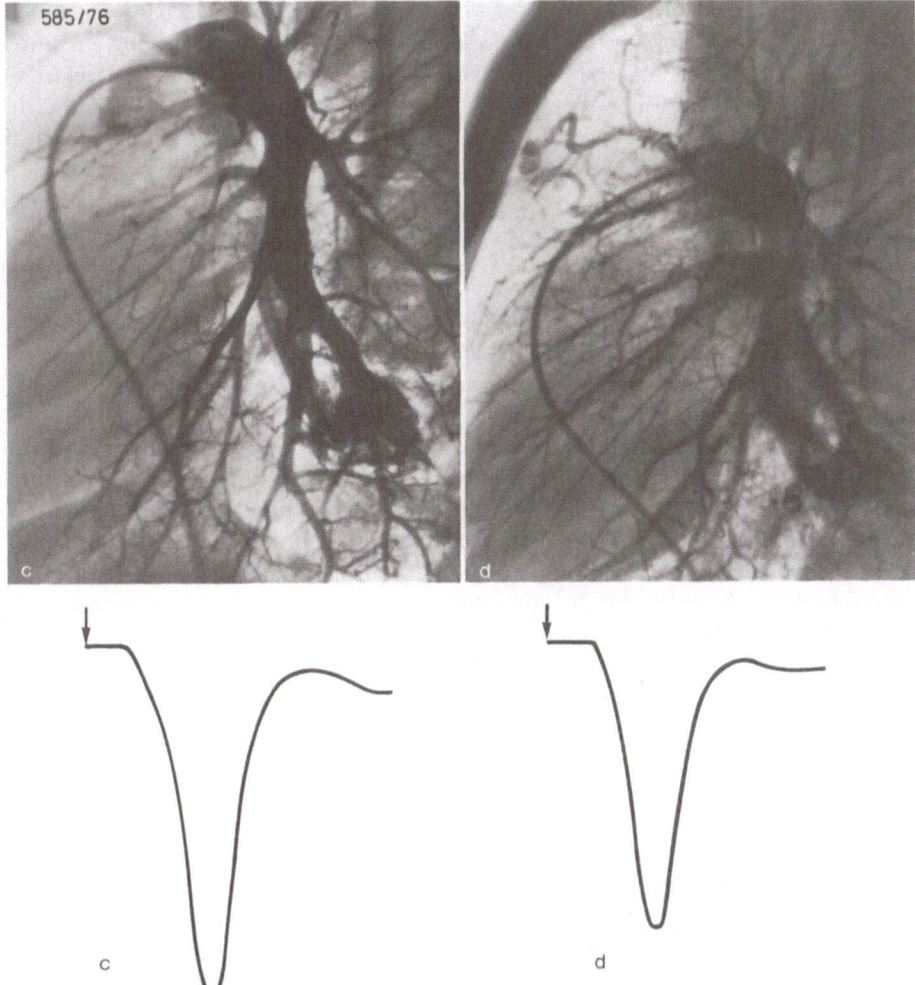

Fig. 2c and d. c) Slight enlargement of the shunt seven months later. Laterobasal segmental branches are involved in the supply of the angioma
d) Status after introduction of four Gianturco spirals. Laterobasal segmental branch is occluded, but the posterobasal artery remains open in spite of the spirals. Additional fistulas in the anterior segment of the upper lobe are now seen
Bottom row: Dye dilution curves (inferior vena cava → femoral artery)

ings. Dye dilution studies from the femoral vein to the femoral artery, in parallel with the ear censor show the success achieved by the procedure and represent the decisive parameter for evaluation.

2. Case Histories

Case 1. A four-year-old boy presented with cyanosis, clubbed fingers and a continuous murmur over the upper lobe of the right lung. Plain films of the thorax showed an opacitiy at the base of the right upper lobe. Selective pulmonary angiography demonstrated an angiomatous a–v fistula in the axillary segment of the upper lobe with premature flow into the left atrium (Fig. 1a).

Therapy. After percutaneous catheterisation of the right femoral artery and selective probing of the right anterior segmental branch with a radiopaque catheter (8-French), a 3 cm long Gianturco spiral was implanted in the anterior segmental branch. Flow through the fistula ceased (Fig. 1b).

Course. The murmur and cyanosis ceased immediately. Angiography showed complete blockage of the fistula. After six months the clubbing of the fingers had regressed discernibly.

Case 2. A 14-year-old boy presented with distinct cyanosis and a loud murmur over the basal segment of the left lower lobe. Angiography showed a large angiomatous a–v fistula in the posterior basal segment (Fig. 2a). Through a 12-French Teflon catheter, 20 Ivalon chips ($5 \times 2 \times 2$ mm) were inserted into the dilated afferent artery. Subsequently the murmur and cyanosis disappeared. Left-sided thoracic pain and pleural rub lasted two days after treatment and then subsided. Angiographic control two months later showed a diminution of the angioma, but a slight residual shunt remained (Fig. 2b). Dye dilution also showed a small right-to-left shunt.
Examination after seven months by angiography and dye dilution revealed a moderate increase in the shunt. Additional subsegmental branches were involved in the filling of the fistula (Fig. 2c). At this time four Gianturco spirals were inserted and these occluded a subsegmental branch. The

condition remained constant during the following months. A control angiogram (Fig. 2d) showed the residual shunt and the occluded subsegmental branch, but a small fistula in the anterior upper lobe segment was seen for the first time. A projected third intervention to block the posterobasal lower lobe branch was abandoned, largely because the patient had no complaints and no enlargement of the right-to-left shunt, shown by dye dilution. At the last examination two additional and previously unrecognised small fistulas were found in the right lower lobe and in the middle lobe. The patient remains under supervision.

Case 3. A 13-year-old boy of below-normal growth presented with cyanosis. A loud systolic-diastolic murmur was heard over the right upper lobe. At the age of two he was first diagnosed as having bilateral angiomatous a–v fistulae (Fig. 3a). At that time the left lower lobe and the lingula were excised. Some ten years later there was an incerease in opacity of the right upper lobe and increased cyanosis. Angiography showed widespread angiomatous fistulas in the apical, posterior and anterior segments of the right upper

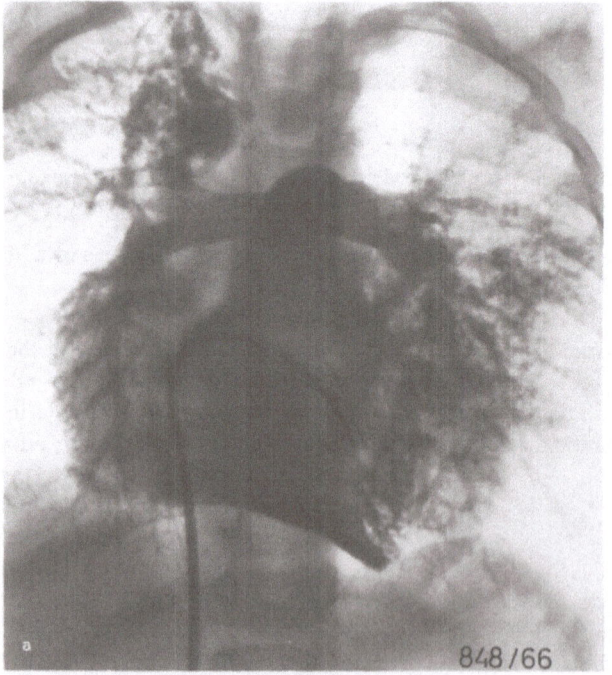

848/66

Fig. 3a–d. Clinical course in multiple bilateral angiomatous a–v fistulas in a boy now 13 years old
a) At two years of age: extensive a–v fistulas in the left lower lobe, lingula, and right upper lobe

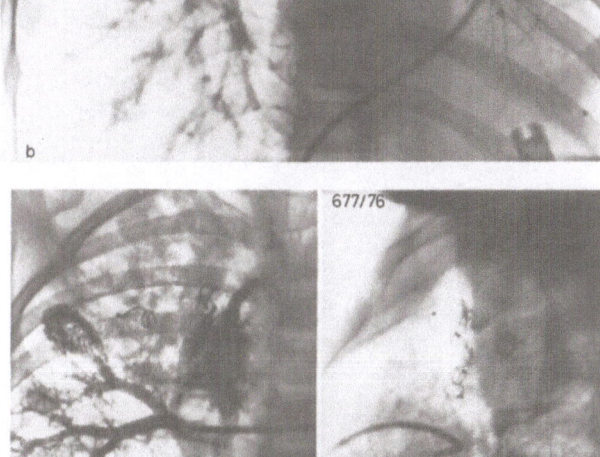

b) Eight years after left-sided bilobectomy with overdistention of the left upper lobe remnant and a small residual fistula. The a–v angioma in the right upper lobe has become increasingly distended

c) Status after treatment of the apical, anterior and (partially) posterior segments of the right upper lobe with six Gianturco spirals
d) Gianturco spirals in the segmental branches of the right upper lobe

lobe (Fig. 3b). Six Gianturco spirals were introduced at two sessions (Fig. 3d). The right-to-left shunt was markedly reduced (Fig. 3c). Clinically, the cyanosis and the murmur have regressed.

Case 4. A 56-year-old woman presented with Osler's disease and a recurrent threatening epistaxis. The chest films showed a walnut-sized coin lesion in the left upper lobe and there was a distinct increase in size over a six-month period. A systolic-diastolic murmur was heard over the left upper lobe. The patient was not cyanotic. Selective pulmonary angiograms showed a typical non-angiomatous a–v pulmonary aneurysm. As a result of the "steal" effect the remaining upper lobe branches were not opacified by contrast medium (Fig. 4a).
Therapy. Two guide wire tips were implanted in the pectoral segmental branch artery through a

percutaneous catheter *(7-French)* introduced into the femoral vein.
Subsequent angiography showed no flow through the a–v aneurysm and the remaining branch arteries of the upper lobe were now opacified (Fig. 4b). At follow-up after one year there was no murmur and on X-ray a marked diminution in size of the coin lesion.

3. Discussion

The aim of the therapeutic catheter procedures discussed in this papier is to block mechanically the main vessels so as to produce ischemia in the subordinate organ (or organ segment). This is-

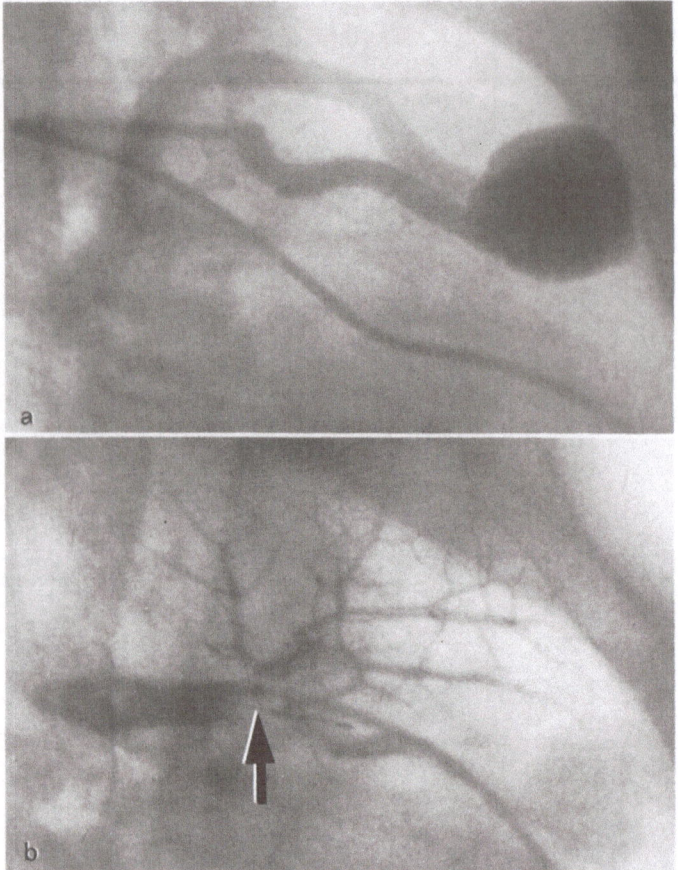

Fig. 4a and b. a). Typical a–v aneurysm in the anterior segment of the upper lobe in a 56-year-old woman
b) Occlusion of the supplying artery after insertion of two guide wire tips (arrow)

chemic state should be irreversible. These procedures *thus* differ fundamentally from catheter procedures in which vasoconstrictive substances are infused to obtain a temporary obstruction of the blood supply to an organ (e.g., in gastrointestinal hemorrhage) [3, 36, 37].

In recent years there has been an increase in clinical case reports describing successful blockage of the arterial circulation employing various catheter techniques. These concern pathologic a–v communications of various kinds, angiomatous tumors or even malignant tumors that are highly vascularized. Many cases are described of intervention in the cerebral circulation [5, 9, 20, 22, 25, 34] and the external carotid artery [16, 17, 26, 40]. Serbinenko [39] reported successful occlusion of post-traumatic carotid sinus fistulas. Angiomatous tumors in the spinal canal have been treated

by embolization [8, 10–12, 28]. In cases of cyanotic heart disease atypical bronchopulmonary communications have been closed by the catheter technique [32, 44]. The occlusion of renal arteries in expansive kidney tumors is finding increasing use [1, 4, 15, 18, 30]. The occlusion of arterial vessels in inoperable tumors of the abdomen or in the pelvis, especially with uncontrollable hemorrhage, have likewise been successfully performed [2, 33, 35, 41, 42]. The occluding materials are introduced by selective direct catheterization of the vessel to be closed or else injected as emboli in the arterial bloodstream in the vicinity of the pathologically vascularized area.

Various substances are employed as occluding material: autologous substances such as clotted blood or muscle pulp [33, 34, 42], aerated plastic foam made of polyvinyl alcohol [18, 30, 31], silicone [12, 16, 27], conducting wire tips and wire spirals with attached wool filaments [14]. Adhesive tissues, with or without radiopaque metal attachments [13, 19, 38, 43] have also been used successfully, experimentally and in humans. This substance can be introduced in liquid form, even through very thin catheters, and it immediately polymerizes on entering the bloodstream; this appears an especially promising development if it proves possible to make it also radiopaque and more readily applicable. In addition, tests are being carried out with infarct-forming radioactive particles [21]. Endovascular electrocoagulation with direct current is at present of only experimental interest. The occurrence of vascular wall necroses debars its use in humans [29].

The elimination of a–v pulmonary fistulas by embolization of the afferent pulmonary artery places special demands on the material to be implanted. The size of the a–v communication is not known in the individual case. Theoretically, if foreign particles that are too small are used there is the danger of embolism in the systemic circulation. Therefore, we prefer to use initially Ivalon chips ($5 \times 2 \times 2$ mm). These, of course, require catheters with wide lumina (10–12-French size), but it is not alway possible to introduce such catheters directly into the vicinity appropriate for embolization. In other cases we have introduced broken-off tips of guide wire into the afferent artery through thin catheters and this has produced thrombus formation. We treated three patients with Gianturco's wire spirals, equipped with wool filaments: when in the catheter they were extended, but they reassumed their spiral form on entering the vessel. In this state they remain absolutely secure in the afferent fistulous vessel. In most cases several spirals (three or four) have to be inserted in order to block the inflow through the dilated artery. On several occasions we found that after eliminating the main flow, we discovered inflow from nearby collateral branches which had previously been unrecognised at angiography. Our present goal is to effect embolization, step-by-step, at several sessions, if it is clinically necessary. Special attention should be paid to multilocular fistulas in order to avoid damage to functionally sound lung tissue.

Two of our four patients were treated at one session, the other two at two sessions. The decision for further embolizations was made on the basis of angiographic control investigations. No complications were observed after the procedures. Only in one case after embolization was there, over a two day period, thoracic pain and a pleural rub. Even when there were residual shunts, there was always an immediate improvment in the hemodynamic status following intervention. In one case, after subtotal occlusion of a large angiomatous fistula, two small fistulas in the other lung were shown on angiography, and previously these had not been demonstrated. These fistulas were certainly not newly formed, but rather fistulas which had escaped detection because of the "steal" effect of the large fistula present at the first study. The so-called "recurrence" (after surgical removal of a fistula or elimination by means of the catheter technique) are more often small fistulas which have been present all the time but have not shown on the initial angiogram.

A comparison between surgical and catheter therapy favours the latter procedure for the following reasons:

1. a thoracotomy is not necessary;
2. in contrast to surgical procedures, the fistula can be eliminated selectively and without affecting functionally sound tissue;
3. since the catheter procedure is selective it is easier to treat multilocular fistulas and this is especially the case when fistulas are bilateral;
4. the lung segment affected remains in situ and so the danger of emphysematous overexpansion of healthy lung segments (which inevitably follows surgical excision) is almost always prevented; and
5. any repeat interventions which may be necessary present no problem, in contrast to surgical procedures.

An immediate repeat intervention is not indicated in every case of incomplete closure or when further fistulas are detected in the course of time. Careful clinical surveillance and selective dye dilution and pulmonary angiographic studies will indicate the right time for any repeat intervention. This is also true for patients previously treated by surgery. When, after the initial treatment, multifocal involvement is apparent then special attention has to be given to the residual smaller fistulas.

4. Summary

Arteriovenous pulmonary fistulas with large right-to-left shunts lead to clear and unequivocal clinical features and may have serious complications. In place of the usual surgical treatment, namely lobectomy, therapeutic embolization of the afferent fistulous artery after selective catheterization is recommended. Substances that will not pass into the systemic circulation are used as embolizing material. Macroparticles made of Ivalon may be used, but wire spirals, which can be localized precisely, have proved especially especially reliable. Details are presented of four patients — three children and one adult — who had uni- or multilocular and bilateral involvement. Their fistulas were treated in one or more stages by the catheter technique. The results of treatment were controlled by angiography. In two cases, closure was total; in the other two, subtotal. The clinical symptoms regressed or were favourably modified. There were no complications.

References

1. ALMGARD, L. E., FERNSTRÖM, I., HAVERLING, M., LJUNGQVIST, A.: Treatment of renal adenocarcinoma by embolic occlusion of the renal circulation. Brit. J. Urol. **45**, 474 (1973)
2. AUNE, S., SCHISTAD, G.: Carcinoid livermetastases treated with hepatic dearterialization. Amer. J. Surg. **123**, 715 (1972)
3. BAUM, S., NUSBAUM, M.: The control of gastrointestinal haemorrhage by selective mesenteric arterial infusion of vasopressin. Radiology **98**, 497 (1971)
4. BOOKSTEIN, J. J., GOLDSTEIN, H. M.: Successful management of post biopsy arteriovenous fistula with selective arterial embolization. Radiology **109**, 535 (1973)
5. CARES, H. L., HALE, J. R., MONTGOMERY, D. B., RICHTER, A. A., SWEET, W.: Laboratory experience with a magnetically guided intravascular catheter system. J. Neurosurg. **38**, 145 (1973)
6. DJINDJIAN, R., COPHIGNON, J., THERON, J., MERLAND, J. J., HOUDART, R.: L'embolisation en neuroradiologie vasculaire. Technique et indications a propos de 30 cas. Presse méd. **1**, 2153 (1972)
7. DJINDJIAN, R., COPHIGNON, J., THERON, J., MERLAND, J. J., HOUDART, R.: Embolization by superselective arteriography from the femoral route in neuroradiology. I Technique, indications, complications. Neuroradiol. **6**, 20 (1973)
8. DJINDJIAN, R., COPHIGNON, J., REY, A., THERON, J., MERLAND, J. J., HOUDART, R.: Superselective arteriographic embolization by the femoral route in neuroradiology. Study of 50 cases. II. Embolization in vertebromedullary pathology. Neuroradiol. **6**, 143 (1973)
9. DJINDJIAN, R., COPHIGNON, J., REY, A., THERON, J., MERLAND, J. J., HOUDART, R.: Superselective arteriographic embolization by the femoral route in neuroradiology. Study of 50 cases. III. Embolization in craniocerebral pathology. Neuroradiol. **6**, 143 (1973)
10. DOPPMAN, J. L., DICHIRO, G., OMMAYA, A.: Obliteration of spinal-cord arteriovenous malformation by percutanoeous embolization. Lancet 1968/ I, 477
11. DOPPMAN, J. L., DICHIRO, G., OMMAYA, A. K.: Percutaneous embolization of spinal cord arteriovenous malformations. J. Neurosurg. **34**, 48 (1971)
12. DOPPMAN, J. L., ZAPOL, W., PIERCE, J.: Transcatheter embolization with a silicone rubber preparation. Experimental observations. Invest. Radiol. **6**, 304 (1971)
13. DOTTER, C. T., GOLDMAN, M. L., RÖSCH, J.: Instant selective arterial occlusion with isobutyl 2-cyanacrylate. Radiology **114**, 227 (1975)
14. GIANTURCO, C., ANDERSON, J. H., WALLACE, S.: Mechanical devises for arterial occlusion. Amer. J. Roentgenol. **124**, 428 (1975)
15. GOLDSTEIN, H. M., MEDELLIN, H., BEN-MENACHEM, Y., WALLACE, S.: Transcatheter arterial embolization in the management of bleeding in the cancer patient. Radiology **115**, 603 (1975)
16. HILAL, S., MOUNT, L., CORREL, J.: Therapeutic embolization of vascular malformations of the external carotid circulation. Clinical and experimental results. IX Symposium Neuroradiologicum, Göteborg, Sweden, Aug. 24—29 (1970)
17. HILAL, S. K., MICHELSON, J. W.: Therapeutic percutaneous embolization for extra-axial vascular lesions of the head, neck and spine. Neurosurg. **43**, 275 (1975)
18. HLAVA, A., STEINHART, L.: Intraluminal obliteration of the renal artery in hypernephroma. Meeting of Czechoslovak. Ass. Radiol., Brunn, 1972
19. KERBER, C.: Experimental arteriovenous fistula creation and percutaneous catheter obstruction with cyanoacrylate. Invest. Radiol. **10**, 10 (1975)
20. KRICHEFF, I. I., MADAYAG, M., BRAUNSTEIN, P.: Transfemoral catheter embolization of cerebral and posterior fossa arteriovenous malformation. Radiology **103**, 107 (1972)
21. LANG, E. K.: Superselective arterial catheterization as a vehicle for delivering radioactive infarctparticles to tumours. Radiology **98**, 391 (1971)

22. LUESSENHOP, A. J., GIBBS, M., VELASQUEZ, A. C.:
Cerebrovascular response to emboli. Observations
in patients with arteriovenous malformations.
Arch. Neurol. **7**, 264 (1962)

23. LUESSENHOP, A. J., KACHMANN, R., JR., SHEV-
LIN, W., FERRERO, A. A.: Clinical evaluation of artificial embolization in the management of large cerebral arteriovenous malformations. J. Neurosurg.
23, 400 (1965)

24. LUESSENHOP, A. J., SPENCE, W. T.: Artificial embolization of cerebral arteries. Report of use in a case
of arteriovenous malformation JAMA **172**, 1153
(1969)

25. LUESSENHOP, A. J., VELASQUEZ, A. C.: Observations
on the tolerance of the intracranial arteries to
catheterization. J. Neurosurg. **21**, 85 (1964)

26. MANELFE, C., GUIRAD, B., DAVID, J., EYMERI, J. C.,
TREMOULET, M., ESPAGNO, J., RASCOL, A., GER-
AUD, J.: Embolisation par cathétérisme des menin-
giomes intracranions. Rev. Neurol. **128**, 339 (1973)

27. MOSSO, J. A., RAND, R. W.: Ferromagnetic silicone
vascular occlusion a technique for selective infarc-
tion of tumours and other organs. Ann. Surg. **178**,
663 (1973)

28. NEWTON, T. H., ADAMS, J. E.: Angiographic demonstration and nonsurgical embolization of
spinal cordangioma. Radiology **91**, 873 (1968)

29. PHILLIPS, J. F.: Transcatheter electrocoagulation of
blood vessels. Invest. Radiol. **8**, 295 (1973)

30. PORSTMANN, W., MÜNSTER, W., FUTH, M., KREBS,
W., SCHWOZER, A.: Die präoperative Embolisation
der Nierenarterie bei malignen Nierentumoren.
Z. Urol. **70**, 165 (1977)

31. PORSTMANN, W., WIERNY, L., WARNKE, H., GERST-
BERGER, G., ROMANIUK, P.: Catheter closure of pat-
ent ductus arteriosus. 62 cases treated without thoracotomy. Radiol. Clin. N. Amer. **9**, 203 (1972)

32. REMY, J., VOISIN, C., DUPUIS, C., BEGENRY, P., TON-
NEL, A. B., DENIES, J. L., DONAY, B.: Treatment of
haemoptysis by embolization of systemic circulation. Ann. Radiol. **17**, 5 (1974)

33. REUTER, S. R., CHUANG, V. P.: Control of abdominal bleeding with autogenous embolized material.
Radiologe **14**, 603 (1968)

34. ROBLES, C., CARRASCO-ZANINI, J.: Treatment of cerebral arterio venous malformations by muscle
embolization. J. Neurosurg. **29**, 603 (1968)

35. RÖSCH, J., DOTTER, C. T., BROWN, M. J.: Selective
arterial embolization. A new method for control of
acute gastrointestinal bleeding. Radiology **102**, 303
(1972)

36. RÖSCH, J., DOTTER, C. T., ANTONOVIC, R.: Selective
vasoconstrictor infusion in the management of ar-
terio-capillary   gastrointestinal   haemorrhage.
Amer. J. Roentgenol. **116**, 279 (1972)

37. RÖSCH, J., DOTTER, C. T., ROSE, R. W.: Selective arterial infusion of vasoconstrictors in acute gastrointestinal bleeding. Radiology **99**, 27 (1971)

38. SANO, K., JINBO, M., SAIRO, I., TORAS, H., HIRAKA-
WA, K.: Artificial embolization with liquid plastic.
Neurol. Medicochir. **8**, 198 (1966)

39. SERBINENKO, F. A.: Kateterizatsiia i okkliuzia mag-
istral 'nykh sosudov golovnogo mozga i perspek-
tivy razvitia sosudistoi neirokhirurgii Vopr. Neiro-
chirur. **35**, 17 (1971)

40. SOKOLOFF, J., WICKBOM, I., MCDONALD, D.: Therapeutic percutaneous embolization in intractible
epistaxis. Radiology **111**, 13 (1974)

41. TADAVARTHY, S. M., KNIGH, L., OVITT, T. W.: Therapeutic transcatheter arterial embolization. Radiology **111**, 13 (1974)

42. WHITE, R. I., JR., GIARGIANA, F. A., JR., BELL, W.:
Bleeding duodenal ulcer control. Selective arterial
embolization with autologous blood cloth.
J.A.M.A. **229**, 546 (1974)

43. ZANETTI, P. H., SHERMAN, F. E.: Experimental evaluation of a tissue adhesive as an agent for the
treatment of aneurysms and arteriovenous anomalies. J. Neurosurg. **36**, 72 (1972)

44. ZUBERBUHLER, J. R., DANKNER, E., ZOLTUN, R.,
BURKHOLDER, J., BAHNSON, T.: Tissue adhesive
closure of aortic-pulmonary communications.
Amer. Heart J. **88**, 41 (1974)

Pediatric Gastrointestinal Fiberendoscopy

N. Cremer, S. Cadranel, P. Rodesch, and M. Cremer

1. Introduction

Fiberoptic endoscopy is now a routine procedure in the diagnosis and treatment of gastrointestinal disease. Roentgenological examination, in spite of recent refinements, may fail to demonstrate certain mucosal lesions.

Pediatric gastroenterology as advanced rapidly in the past few decades and so have the concomitant endoscopic procedures. Adequate miniaturized fiberoptic instruments have added a new dimension to endoscopy in paediatric gastroenterology. Such fiberoptic endoscopies can now be performed routinely in children without general anaesthesia.

The purpose of this survey of fiberoptic endoscopy in children is to give a contemporary account of the instruments, techniques and the specific information which is derived from and which is distinctive to fiberoptic endoscopy.

2. Instruments

In the late sixties, although endoscopy acquired widespread popularity, the only instruments available were of large caliber. These were not suitable for use in children, except for bronchofiberscopes which are only appropriate to study of the respiratory tract.

The first prototype of the paediatric instrument for study of the alimentary tract became available in 1972. Subsequent developments in instruments have made it possible to perform panendoscopy in children and in infants.

Optical Characteristics. In fiberoptic endoscopes the quality of the picture is related directly to the number and quality of glass fibres. Paediatric instruments, for use either in the alimentary tract or respiratory tract, are thinner and so the number of glass fibres is less and quality of the image is reduced when compared to that in instruments in use in adult work.

Mechanical Characteristics. Instruments designed for use in adult gastroenterology have distinctive characteristics, namely, a four way bending of the tip, a large biopsy channel, a push button system for in and out circulation of air, and a facility for washing the lens. It is difficult to design a miniaturized instrument with all these capabilities. Miniaturization has often been accompanied by loss of the capacity to bend in one plane—allowing only two ways bending.

For paediatric fiberendoscopy to be acceptable thin fiberscopes are essential. Currently, there are five instruments which have been designed specifically for the paediatric age range. The instruments are:

1. The Olympus PFG-S (paediatric gastrofiberscope) permits lateral viewing and is the thinnest (5 mm). However, it is not equipped with a biopsy channel and it has no suction system. The air and water insufflation system is not automatic and it is inefficient. The flexible bending tip is too short and this makes it difficult to pass the instrument into the antrum.

2. The GIF-P (pediatric gastrointestinal fiberscope) has a 7.2 mm diameter and permits frontal viewing. This instrument is the first commercially available endoscope which is really useful in children. The caliber is thin enough to permit study of both infants and children. However, the

French 5 gauge biopsy forceps tends to be hampered by friction in passing along the instrument and the biopsy samples (1cu mm) are often too small to permit a complete pathological analysis. Nevertheless, the push button system for washing the lens and the air circulation are both satisfactory. The bending segment of the tip is a little too long and it moves only in one plane, but with experience rotation of the instrument can be used to countervail this limitation: this enables progress from the stomach, through the pylorus and into the duodenum to be made. Since the tip does not bend sufficiently there are areas which cannot be viewed by the instrument in transit.

3. The Olympus prototypes JF-D and JF-D 1000 are somewhat larger (8.2 mm) and permit forward viewing. The tip can be bent in all directions. These instruments are preferable for paediatric fiberendoscopy except for infants of less than 3 months. The biopsy forceps (French 5 gauge) pass easily through the channel.

The improved bending characteristics of the tip reduce the extent of the areas which are not seen. These instruments are more fragile but, because they are more flexible, they are better tolerated by patients. They may be used for colonoscopy, provided adequate sterilization is available [1].

4. The ACMI-F7 is a recently developed instrument. It has a 9.5 mm diameter, forward viewing and it is polydirectional.

It is a little too large for children under 4 years of age. The larger bending angle makes it easier to manipulate for someone who is used to the "two hand-knob" system. However, this unit's optical systems seem to be inferior to those of the Olympus systems.

5. The JF-B2 duodenoscope has lateral viewing, a diameter of 10 mm, and it can be used without difficulty in children of school age.

6. The new polydirectional fiberscope GIF-P2 has an 8.5 mm diameter. It has thin fibers and these give fine resolution in the round image. These features make it among the very best developed in the most recent times and it surely points to the future trends in development.

The larger conventional fiberscopes can be used in teenagers without any need for anaesthesia.

For colonoscopy it is advisable to use only forward viewing instruments. In colonooscopy caliber is less important and standard colonscopes can be used, if necessary, in children over 4 years of age. However, a miniaturized endoscope is preferable, because it permits an examination which is free of pain. Although in colonoscopy four directions of tip bending are helpful, satisfactory examinations as far as the ileo-caecal valve are entirely possible with the two directional bending tips of the GJF-P.

For rectosigmoidoscopy the fiberscope makes the examination more comfortable for the patient and it also gives more reliable diagnostic results than rigid instruments: The rigid proctoscope and sigmoidoscope no longer have a place in the examination of children.

The sterilization of fiberscopes is important and we use the method described by AXON and co-workers [1]: this method gives protection for patients and yet preserves the instruments.

Cold light supply sources which are appropriate are the Olympus CLE 111 (halogen 150 W bulb), the Sass-Wolf Endoblitz (halogen 150 W bulb) with a special flash bulb and the Olympus CLX (Xenon 300 W bulb). Because of the physiological tachypnea of children, sharp pictures can only be obtained with a fast shutter speed on the camera, and this means a flash unit must be used.

3. Preparation and Premedication

For upper gastrointestinal endoscopy 4 to 8 h fasting is necessary. In children under 6 years of age local analgesia of the throat must not be carried out with the standard commercially available sprays because these have too high a concentration of lidocaine (Xylocaine R) and one spray delivers 10 mgm.

Fasting is not required for colonoscopy, but a perfect cleaning of the colon is essential. This can be achieved by giving the child a low residue diet for 3 days and isotonic enemas each day.

Anaesthesia is required only if adult type fiberscopes are used in small children. The examination can be carried out in children with sedation only if miniaturized fiberscopes are used. In infants nembutal (8 mgm/Kg of body weight) and in children pethidine (2 mgm/Kg of body weight) give the best results. When upper gastrointestinal examinations are carried out atropine (0.01 mgm/Kg body weight) is given simultaneously. Passing the fiberscope through the duodenum may sometimes prove difficult when atropine has been given too early and so it is best to examine the duodenum first.

A good psychological preparation is always more helpful than any medication and allows follow-up studies to be performed without undue reluctance on the part of the child.

4. Training

It takes at least two years' training to be able to perform all kinds of endoscopic examinations.

There are two problems which the beginner encounters. The first is that of becoming familiar with handling and manoevring the instrument. The second is that of recognising lesions and appreciating their significance. It is therefore best to acquire training in a large center for endoscopy where an organised teaching programme is in existence.

5. Indications and Findings [2, 4, 5]

Fiberoptic endoscopy is a safe procedure and we have encountered no complications in 620 examinations carried out in children whose ages have ranged from 10 days to 16 years.

The medical indications for fiberoptic endoscopy are summarized in Figure 1: these details derive

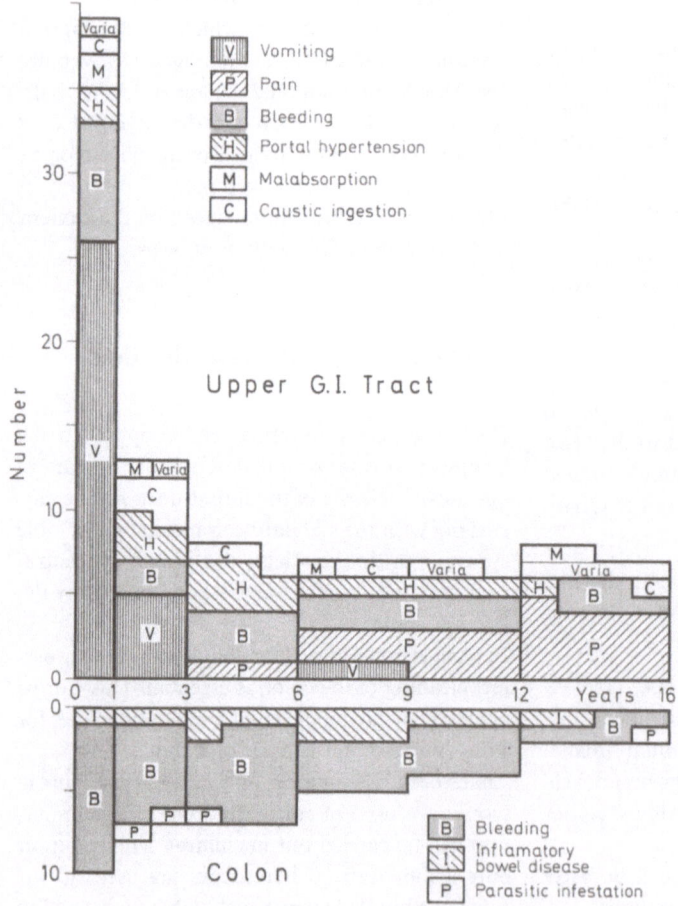

Fig. 1. The indications for U.G.I. endoscopies and colonoscopies according to the different age groups

from the first 400 cases studied. Since this first series additional cases have not changed the emphasis among indications.

Upper Gastrointestinal Tract [3, 6, 7, 9, 15]. Gastrointestinal bleeding is an important reason for fiberoptic endoscopy in a child of any age. Persistent vomiting in infants and epigastric pain mainly in school children are also important indications for this study. Oesophagoscopy is always carried out when portal hypertension is suspected or if caustics have been ingested: together these indications represent a major fraction of the total. The endoscopist can easily recognise minimal alterations of the mucosa such as colour change and slight oedema. Oesophagitis (Fig. 2)[1] represents 30% and gastritis 24% of the positive findings. However, it must be emphasized that these endoscopic findings of "oesophagitis" and "gastritis" were not always checked by a conclusive pathological study.

The areae gastricae are very often demonstrated by a radiological double contrast technique or with a high KV and fluid barium technique: they need special care to be detected during a routine gastroscopy, but are easier to identify when dye (such as Evans blue) is injected onto the surface. Pseudopolypoid gastritis, even if localized, can be detected by radiology as well as by endoscopy (Figs. 5, 6, 7).

The remainder of the findings comprised oesophageal varices 14% (Figs. 3, 4) duodenitis 9%, gastro-duodenal ulcers 9%, pyloric stenosis 6%, and duodenal stenosis 2%.

Radiological investigations have been performed first, exempting when bleeding is occurring. Radiology failed to show superficial oesophagitis (Fig. 2), varices less severe than grade 2 or grade 3, acute haemorrhagic gastritis and some superficial ulcers (Fig. 9).

When a superficial ulcer is greater than 2 mm diameter it can be demonstrated by a double contrast radiological technique (Fig. 8). However, the indications for this technique are less frequently encountered than in adults and so it is not so widely practised and generally children do not accept the necessary sophisticated preparation quite so well. In any event, when bleeding is occurring

---

[1] Figures 2, 3, 6, 7, 9, 12, 13, 15–17 have been placed together as a table on p. 36

the radiologist can never be certain that any lesion he demonstrates is the source of bleeding.

Many children have multiple or associated lesions. Therefore, when a child is bleeding, endoscopy must be performed as soon as possible and within 12 h: this increases the chance of finding the causative lesion. Most of these lesions are acute tiny superficial ulcers which disappear in a few days (Fig. 9). Since the advent of fiberoptic endoscopy, it is our experience that the number of demonstrable ulcers has increased.

Barium swallow and meal techniques are better than endoscopy for studying general structure, relationships, and motility.

Endoscopic Retrograde Cholangiopancreatography (ERCP). In childhood ERCP is performed under general anaesthesia. The indications are obstructive jaundice, jaundice of unknown origin and pancreatic disease. The frequency with which ERCP is performed in children is lower than in adults.

The diagnostic value of this technique is unquestionable. Five patients have been studied by ERCP. The biliary tract and main pancreatic duct were normal in one patient. Two cases of chronic pancreatitis were demonstrated. In a case of Schwachman disease an atretic pancreatic duct was found. A stenosis of the biliary duct was shown in the fifth case (Fig. 10).

Colonoscopy [13]. The length and multiple flexures of the colon often mean that colonoscopy is difficult and it can take a long time. In general, colonoscopy has proved most useful in the diagnosis of rectal bleeding, inflammatory bowel disease and (in adults) the early diagnosis of cancer. In both infants and children rectal bleeding has been by far the most common indication for colonoscopy. Juvenile polyps accounts for 35% of positive findings in our series. Non-specific colitis constitutes a further 20%. Chronic inflammatory changes of ulcerative colitis or Crohn's disease represent a total of 17%. Other conditions have a minor incidence—parasitic infestations 5%, trauma 7%, ulcero-necrotic colitis 2% and angiomatosis 4%.

Barium enema failed to demonstrate polyps subsequently shown by endoscopy because of unsatisfactory preparation and cleansing of the bowel.

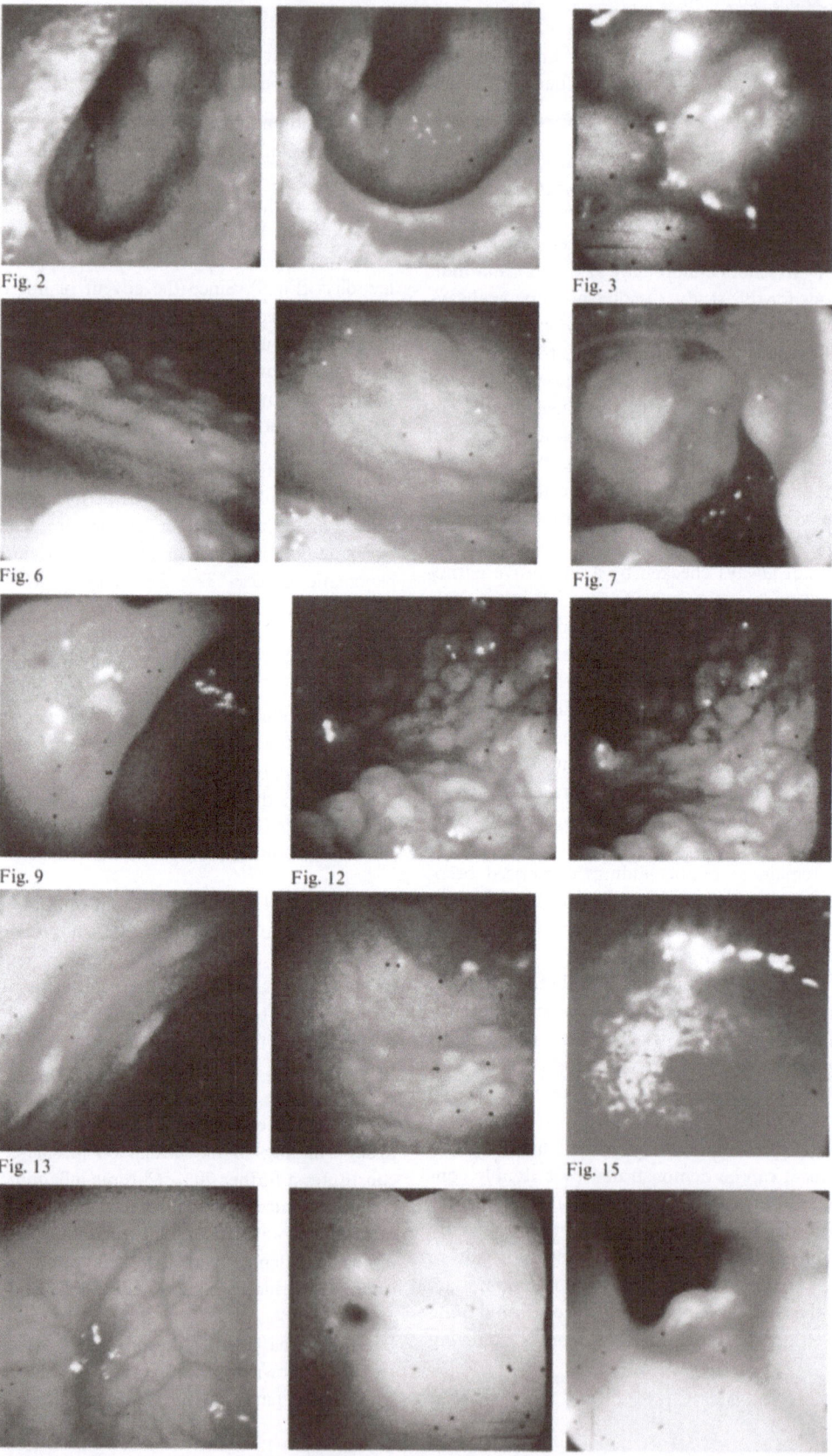

Fig. 2

Fig. 3

Fig. 6

Fig. 7

Fig. 9

Fig. 12

Fig. 13

Fig. 15

Fig. 16

Fig. 17

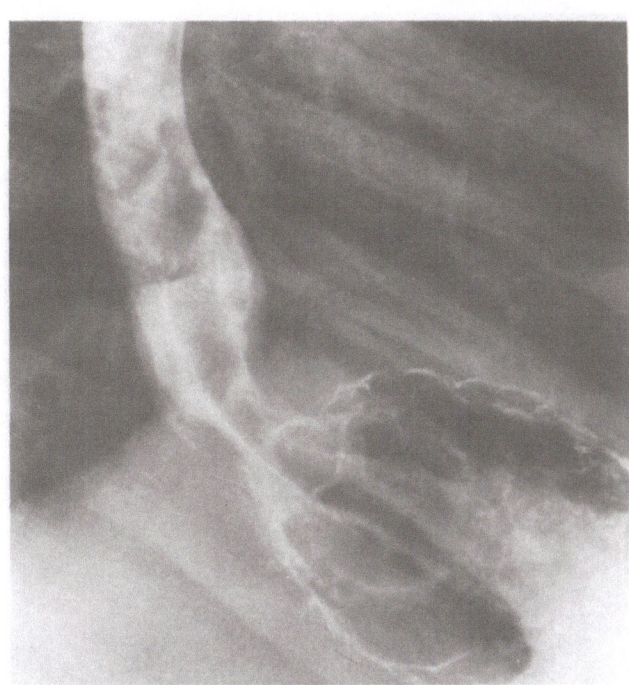

Fig. 4. 2½ year old boy. Esophageal varices grade 2. The varix looks like a big longitudinal fold

Polyps located in any site of the colon can be resected at endoscopy and then pathological studies carried out. Barium enema examination is, by comparison with endoscopy, a less reliable and distinctly limited investigatory technique.

In general the correlation between radiology and endoscopy in evaluating inflammatory diseases has been excellent (Figs. 11, 12), for example, in Crohn's disease and ulcerative colitis. The exceptions have been two cases of ulcerative colitis where the barium enema was misleadingly normal and one case of Crohn's disease where the extent of the anatomical lesion could not be evaluated by colonoscopy because the fiberscope could not be passed sufficiently far into the gut.

Endoscopy in cases of so-called lymphoid hyperplasia shows small scattered polypoid formations with a little jelly-like material at the apex of each polyp (Fig. 13). The central umbilication seen in the polypoid-like images in the lymphoid hyperplasia at barium enema are not visible at endoscopy (Fig. 14).

The most cautious interpretation must be given to minimal changes of the mucosa when there is no

---

Fig. 2. Esophagitis in a case of hiatal hernia (18 months). Reddened swollen mucosa and pseudomembranes

Fig. 3. Endoscopic view of esophageal varices in a 3½ years old boy. The varices have a blue colour

Fig. 6. Endoscopic view of the polypoid formation. Same Case as Fig. 5

Fig. 7. Polypoid formation in gastritis in a 10 year old girl

Fig. 9. Small superficial ulcer of the antrum in a 4 year old boy missed at X-ray investigations

Fig. 12. Same case as Figure 11. Pseudopolypoid formation at endoscopy

Fig. 13. Endoscopic view in "lymphoid hyperplasia"— small scattered minute polypoid structures

Fig. 15. A case of amoebic colitis in a 2½ year old girl showing a bleeding mucosa with depressions. Radiological findings were those of "lymphoid hyperplasia"

Fig. 16. Colonic angioma

Fig. 17. Esophageal stenosis in a 2 year old boy before and after endoscopic dilatation

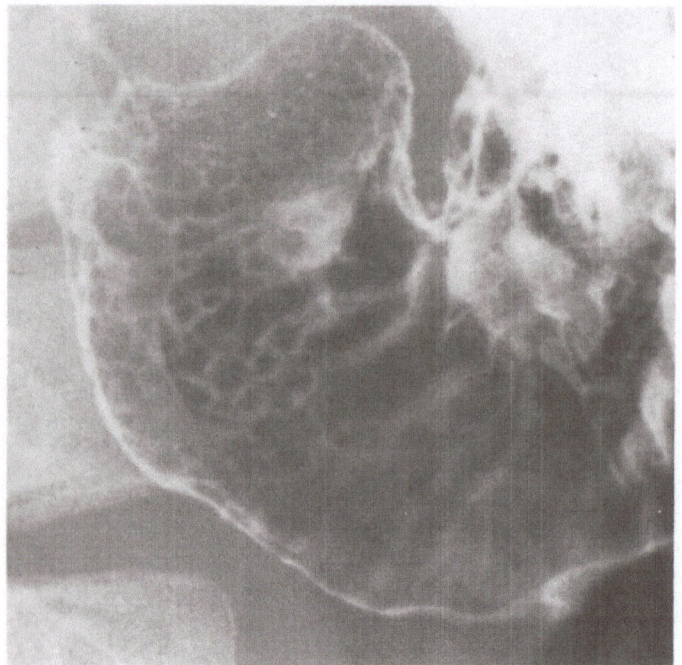

Fig. 5. 9 year old girl. Polypoid gastritis limited to the antrum

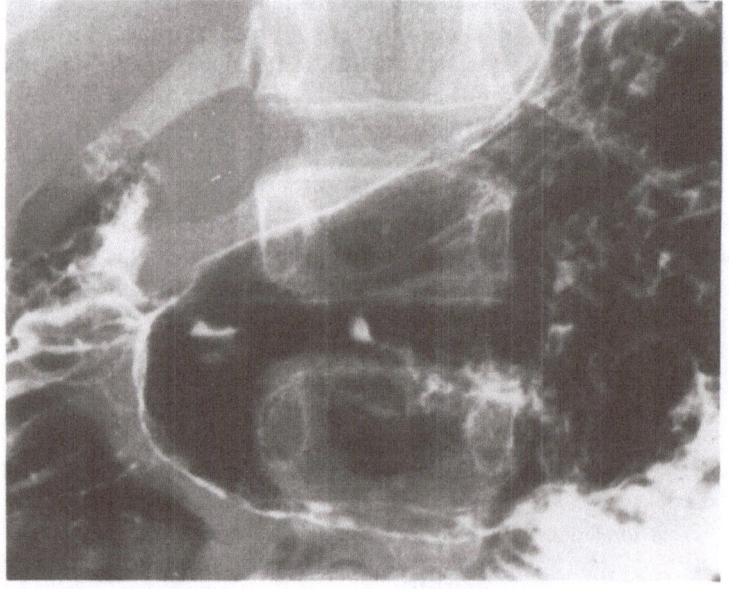

Fig. 8. Two superficial ulcers located in the antrum in a 11 year old girl (double contrast technique)

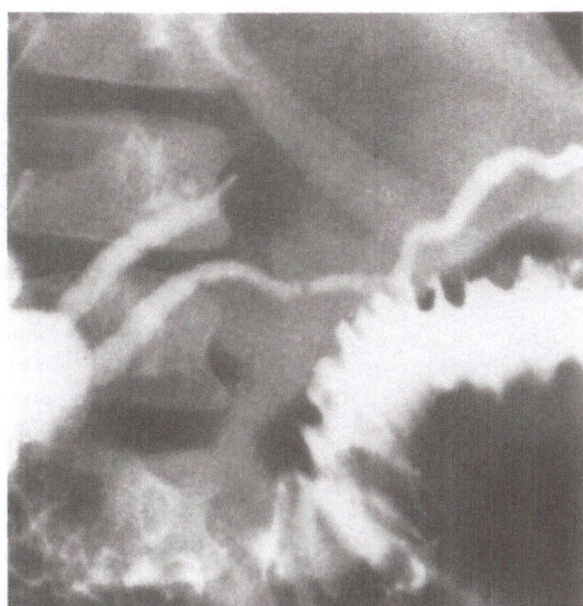

Fig. 10. E.R.C.P. Stenosis of the biliary duct in a $3^1/_3$ year old boy. Normal duct of Wirsung

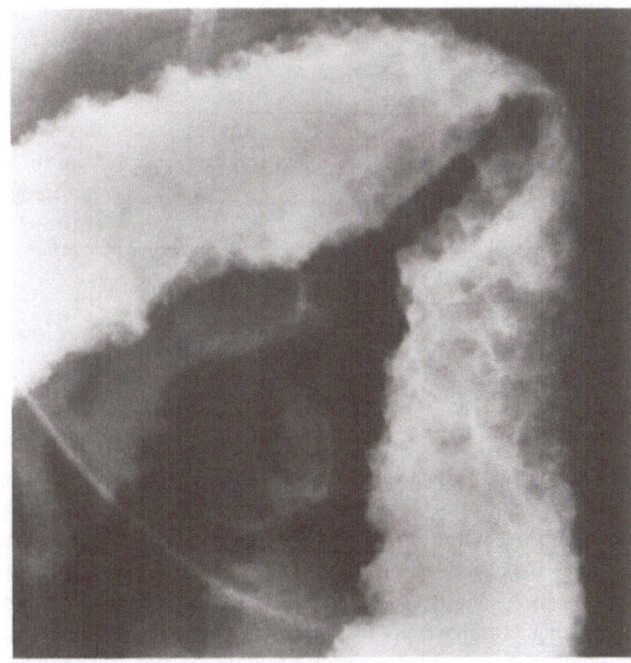

Fig. 11. Ulcerative colitis in a 9 year old girl

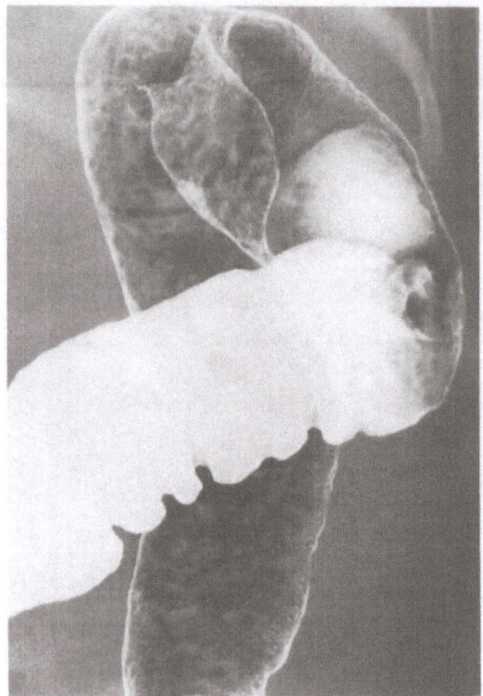

Fig. 14. Radiological features of colonic "lymphoid hyperplasia"

colour alteration. However, Figure 15 shows the features at endoscopy in amoebic colitis.

Multiple biopsies taken under direct vision at endoscopy show only non-specific inflammatory changes.

Angiomas may be seen at endoscopy when they are not visible on barium enema (Fig. 16).

6. Therapeutic Aspects of Endoscopy

1. Foreign Body Removal [11, 14]. In radiology the identification of a foreign body is related to the atomic weight of material in the foreign body. However, the endoscopist is able to detect all types of foreign body of any size.

Removing a foreign body from the oesophagus is possible with a forward viewing paediatric fiberscope. When a foreign body is in the stomach it is often easier to use a lateral viewing conventional JFBR and a wire loop in a 5 French gauge cath-

eter. General anaesthesia can be advantageous for removing foreign bodies for then standard models of fiberscopes can be used with all their accessories and a 7 French gauge channel.

2. Oesophageal Dilatation [12]. Fiberoptic endoscopy is particularly useful in treating oesophageal strictures. Classically dilatation has been achieved by rubber bougies. However, with endoscopy it is possible to use the Eder-Pustow technique. Steel olives are introduced on a wire guide previously passed through the stenosis under endoscopic control. This technique reduces the risk of perforation especially when the stenosis is eccentric: nevertheless there is the risk of perforation when the stenosis is long and caused by caustic oesophagitis.

In children, dilatation relieves the symptoms of an oesophageal stricture and this can avoid gastrostomy and sometimes the need for surgery (Fig. 17, 18). Three peptic stenoses have been cured, but a child with persistent reflux needed operation. In two cases with caustic strictures perforation occurred when dilatation of the lower part of the stenoses was carried out.

3. Polypectomy [16]. Juvenile polyps are most often located in the rectosigmoid: these polyps are more easily removed through the colonoscope than through a rigid sigmoidoscope. At fiberoptic endoscopy resection is performed with a diathermy loop.

7. Conclusion

With appropriate instruments and in skilled hands fiberoptic endoscopy is a safe and valuable procedure in investigating the gastrointestinal tract. It is usually possible to perform the procedure without anaesthesia and yet make the investigation reasonably comfortable for the child.

The main indication for endoscopy is bleeding from the gastrointestinal tract.

The fiberendoscope provides an advance in technique when dilating short oesophageal stenoses. The choice between an endoscopic or a radiological type of investigation can sometimes be diffi-

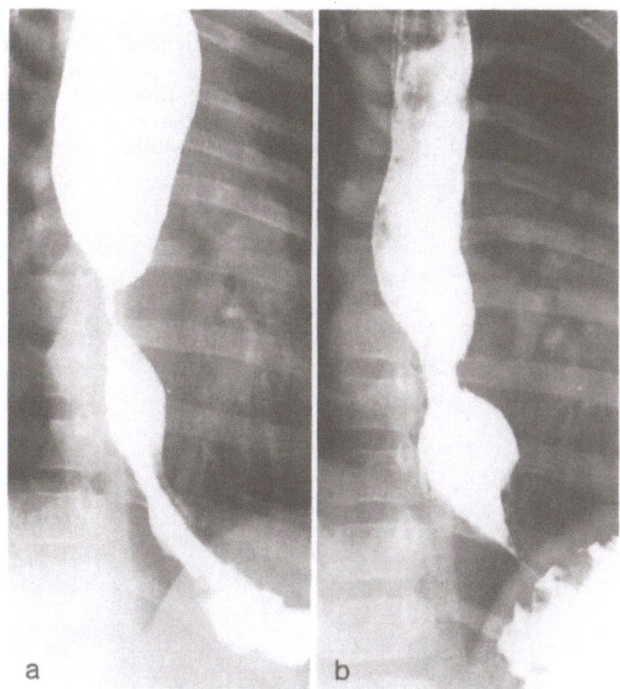

Fig. 18. Endoscopic view of a stenosis
before and after dilatation   a   b

cult. However, when one of these techniques has
given an accurate and complete diagnosis there is
no need to use the other.

References

1. AXON, A. T. R., COTTON, P. B., PHILIPS, I., AVERY,
   S. A.: Desinfection of gastrointestinal fiberendo-
   scopes. Lancet I, 656—658 (1974)
2. CADRANEL, S., RODESCH, P., PEETERS, J. P., CRE-
   MER, M.: Fiberendoscopy of the gastrointestinal
   tract in children: a series of 100 examinations.
   Amer. J. Dis. Child. (under press) (1976)
3. COTTON, P. B.: Fiberoptic endoscopy and the barium meal: results and implications. Brit. Med. J.
   II, 161—165 (1973)
4. CREMER, M.,   PEETERS, J. P.,   EMONTS, P.,   RO-
   DESCH, P., CADRANEL, S.: Fiberendoscopy of the
   gastrointestinal tract in children. Experience with
   newly designed fiberscopes. Endoscopy 6, 186—
   189 (1974)
5. CREMER, M., RODESCH, P., CADRANEL, S.: Progress
   report: Paediatric gastrointestinal fiberendoscopy.
   To be published in GUT
6. FORGET, P. P., MERADJI, M.: Contribution of fiberoptic endoscopy to diagnosis and management of
   children with gastro-esophageal reflux. Arch. Dis.
   Child. 51, 60—66 (1976)
7. FREEMAN, N. V.: Paediatric gastroscopy Lancet I,
   1351 (1971)
8. GLEASON, W. A.,   TEDESCO, F. J.,   KEATING, J. P.,
   GOLDSTEIN, P. D.: Fiberoptic gastrointestinal endoscopy in infants and children. J. Pediat. 85,
   810—813 (1974)
9. MARCHAT, F., MOULINIER, B., DE PRADO, R., LAM-
   BERT, R.: L'oeso-gastro-duodénoscopie en pédiatrie. Acta Endoscopica et Radiocinématographica
   5, 15—21 (1975)
10. MOUGENOT, J. F.,   MONTAGNE, J. PH.,   FAURE, C.:
    Gastrintestinal fibro-endoscopy in infants and
    children: radio-fibroscopic correlations. Ann. Ra-
    diol., 1976 19 (I), 23—24 (1976)
11. OTTENJANN, R.: Gastroscopic extraction of foreign
    body. Endoscopy, 3, 193—194 (1970)
12. PRICE, J. D., STANCHI, C., BENNET, J. R.: A safer
    method of dilating esophageal strictures. Lancet I,
    1141—1142 (1974)
13. RODESCH, P., CADRANEL S., PEETERS, J. P., CRE-
    MER, N., CREMER, M.: Colonic endoscopy in child-
    ren. Acta Paed. Belg. (under press) (1976)

14. ROESCH, W., CLASSEN, M.: Fiberendoscopic foreign body removal from the upper gastrointestinal tract. Endoscopy **4**, 193—197 (1972)

15. VON HENNING, H., SCHMID, E., LOOK, D., MERKEL, W., VON BRAUN, H.H.: Vergleich der Zeichen des Pfortaderhochdrucks im laparoskopischen, ösophagoskopischen und röntgenologischen Bild. Zeitsch. Gastroenterologie **10**, 609—622 (1972)

16. WOLFF, W.I., SHINYA, H.: Polypectomy via the fiberoptic colonoscope. New England Journal of Medecine **288**, 329—332 (1973)

The Esophagus in Infancy

B. R. Girdany

Congenital and acquired lesions of the pharynx and esophagus are important causes of morbidity in infants and children. Cineradiographic and videotape recording of fluoroscopic examinations have added greatly to the understanding of these conditions [2, 5]. In general, lesions of the proximal esophagus and pharynx lead to *aspiration* of mucus or feedings and produce symptoms referable to the respiratory tract. Conditions that affect the mid and distal portion of the esophagus cause *vomiting*.

Fluoroscopic examination of the infant and uncooperative child requires immobilization of the patient. Immobilization shortens the examination, limits irradiation, and affords the radiologist direct control of the examination. The radiologist can satisfactorily evaluate disorders of swallowing by feeding the infant opaque liquids form a bottle. The infant is placed on his back in a left anterior oblique position so that he can be fed comfortably. Direct lateral positioning makes bottle feeding by nipple technically difficult.

The oblique muscle fibers of the inferior constrictors of the pharynx and the transverse fibers of the cricopharyngeus seem to function together in producing *disorders of swallowing* in infancy. It is, therefore, convenient to consider both sets of muscles together as the cricopharyngeus for purposes of discussion.

The obstetrician may damage the posterior pharyngeal wall of an infant during breech delivery, producing a tear in the wall and a traumatic pseudo-diverticulum [4, 6] (Figs. 1 and 2). The infant with traumatic *pseudo-diverticulum* of his posterior pharyngeal wall acts as though he has esophageal atresia; obstruction is caused by crico-pharyngeal spasm or achalasia. Traumatic pseudo-diverticula can occur in older infants and children after trauma to the posterior pharyngeal wall [10]. The newborn infant may develop cricopharyngeal difficulties following attempts to intubate or suction his hypopharynx after delivery or after a difficult birth (Fig. 3). Infants with meningomyeloceles have cricopharyngeal achalasia and so aspirate.

Brain stem tumors may cause swallowing difficulties. Children with the *Riley-Day syndrome* (dysautonomia) characteristically aspirate and do not have normal cough reflexes [9]. In these children, delayed relaxation of the cricopharyngeus is responsible for aspiration. Cricopharyngeal dysfunction causes aspiration of feedings in micrognathic infants. "*Fatigue*" *aspiration* is a recently recognized disorder of swallowing in which affected infants aspirate the terminal portions of large liquid feedings [3]. It is likely that aspiration is due to fatigue of the cricopharyngeus.

Children who swallow lye may develop *cricopharyngeal achalasia* and aspirate liquids (Fig. 4) [2]. Swelling of the epiglottis indicates that the caustic material has reached the hypopharynx and esophagus in significant amounts (Fig. 5).

Esophageal atresia with or without tracheo-esophageal fistula is the most important congenital malformation of the esophagus. It produces early difficulties with swallowing. The diagnosis of esophageal atresia depends on the demonstration of an opaque nasal catheter meeting constant obstruction at the blind end of the infant's proximal esophageal segment [2, 5]. In general, contrast material is not necessary to confirm the diagnosis of esophageal atresia.

Current attention is directed to the complications that follow surgical repair of esophageal atresia. Stenosis at the site of anastomosis results in persistent dilatation of the proximal esophageal segment which impinges on and narrows the tracheal lumen (Fig. 6), causing cough and respiratory dis-

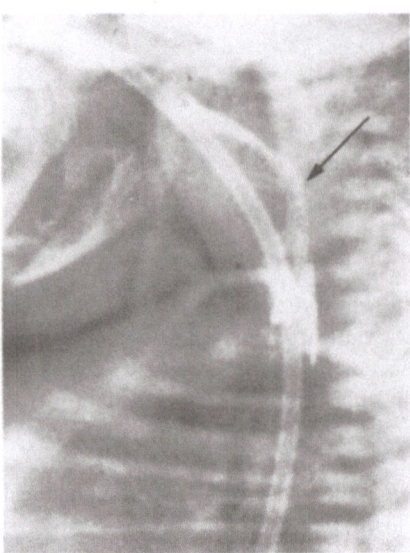

Fig. 1. Lateral view of nasopharynx and chest with nasogastric tube in place in an infant 12 h of age. Opaque
material (*arrow*) lies in traumatic *pseudodiverticulum*
of *pharynx*. Infant was delivered vaginally after breech
presentation. Admitting diagnosis was esophageal
atresia. Attending physician had been unable to pass a
nasogastric tube. Infant was treated without surgery
and was fed by nasogastric tube for 7 days

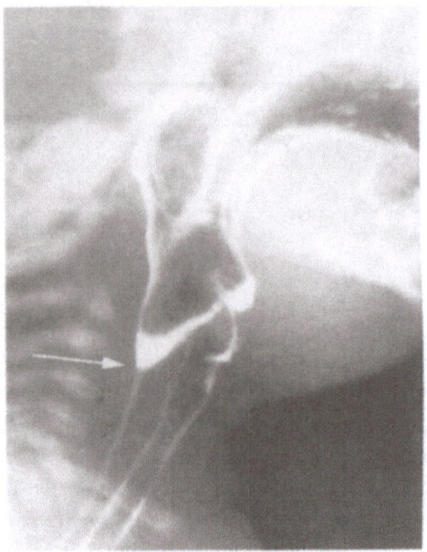

Fig. 3. Lateral view of nasopharynx after barium swallow in a 1-day-old infant who regurgitated milk and
drooled excessively. Cricopharyngeal achalasia and
tracheal aspiration are seen. Right side of infant's face
was swollen. A week later, after treatment with naso-
pharyngeal suction and nasogastric tube feeding, the
infant swallowed normally

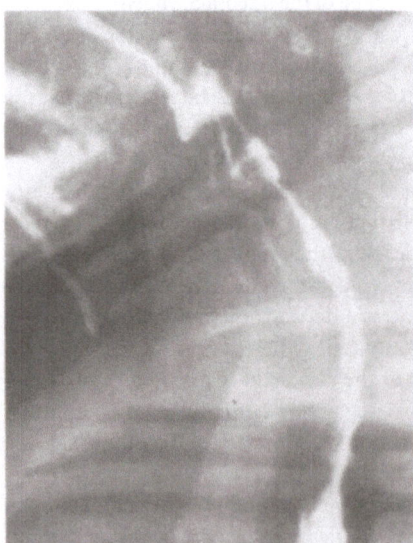

Fig. 2. Lateral esophagram obtained when infant was 8
months of age, doing well, but with some dysphagia.
Esophagram shows evidence of cricopharyngeal achalasia and tracheal aspiration

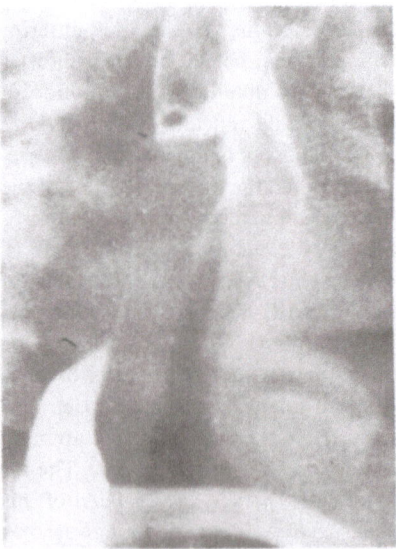

Fig. 4. Lateral film of neck and nasopharynx after barium swallow in a child who had ingested lye 2 weeks
earlier. Proximal segment of cervical esophagus is narrow and barium mixture has been aspirated into the
trachea

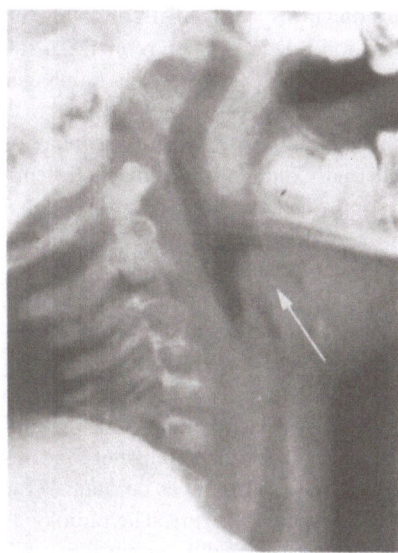

Fig. 5. Lateral film of the same child's nasopharynx, made 20 h after ingestion of lye, shows a swollen epiglottis

tress with feedings. *Recurrent tracheo-esophageal fistula* (Fig. 7) is suspected when respiratory distress, with or without abdominal distention, occurs postoperatively. Occasionally, infants have *congenital stenosis of the esophagus* immediately beyond the level of anastomosis or *hiatus hernias.* These latter may be congenital, or may follow necessary tension on the lower segment of the esophagus during surgical anastomosis of the two ends of the esophagus.

Infants who have had successful surgical repair of esophageal atresia usually have abnormal *motility* in their distal *esophageal* segments. Approximately 10% lack normal peristaltic motility in their upper esophageal segments. Manometric pressure studies and fluoroscopic examination identify abnormal peristalsis [11].

Tracheo-esophageal fistula without esophageal atresia causes respiratory distress often associated with abdominal distention or meteorism (Fig. 8). The same fistula that allows food to enter the

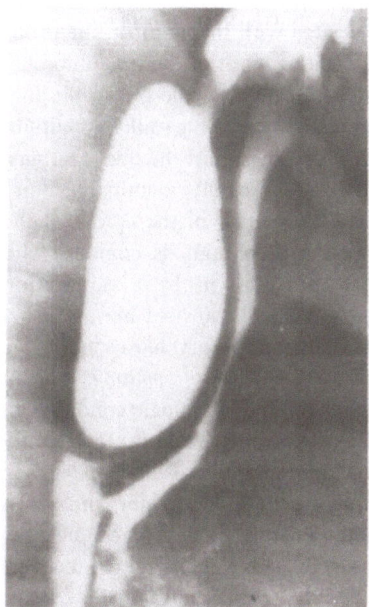

Fig. 6. Barium esophagram after surgical repair of esophageal atresia with tracheoesophageal fistula. Proximal segment of esophagus is distended, overflow aspirations filsla trachea. Distended proximal esophagus compresses trachea from behind, narrowing its lumen. Narrowing at site of esophageal anastomosis is apparent

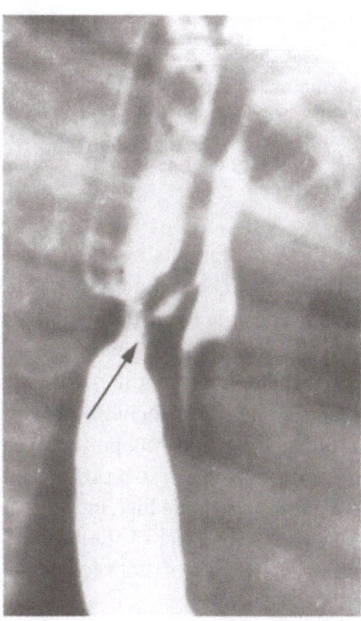

Fig. 7. Recurrent tracheoesophageal fistula between esophagus at the level of primary anastomosis and trachea at original site of fistula

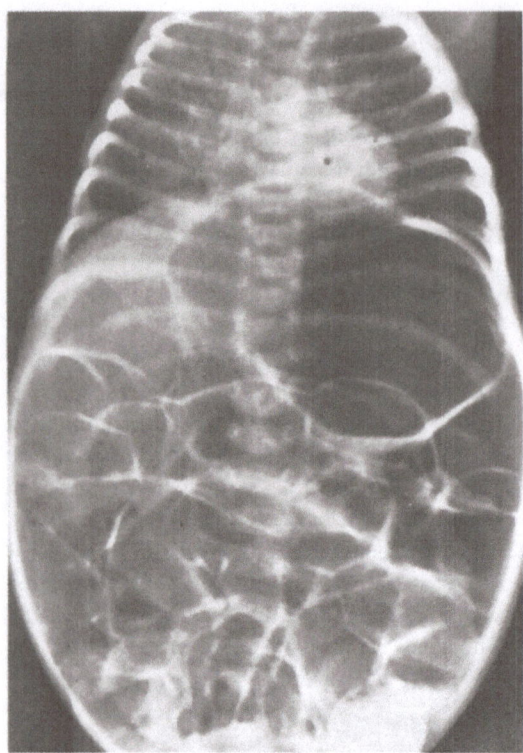

Fig. 8. Gaseous distention of the bowel in a 3-month-old girl with tracheo-esophageal fistula. Lungs show widespread bronchopneumonia. This infant had had repeated bouts of respiratory distress with abdominal distention

lungs may allow massive amounts of air to enter the gastrointestinal tract. The radiologist identifies *tracheo-esophageal fistula* by introducing barium solution into the proximal portion of the infant's esophagus through a nasal tube with the pressure of a hand syringe. He includes the infant's hypopharynx in the fluoroscopic field so that he can differentiate between aspiration and true fistula. Fistulas may originate high in the esophagus, at or just above the level of the bifurcation of the trachea, or from the distal segment of the esophagus [7].

Congenital stenosis of the *esophagus* is a relatively common condition. It may cause high esophageal obstruction, but usually it affects the esophagus at the junction of its distal third and proximal two-thirds [2, 5]. Symptoms in this latter group are recognized after the infant begins a diet of chopped and table foods. The clinician should consider this diagnosis in any infant or child who has impacted food or foreign body in the distal third of the esophagus. Stenosis of the esophagus should not be confused with strictures that may result from or accompany Reflux esophagitis and hiatus hernia. Children with congenital stenosis of the esophagus have normal cardioesophageal junctions.

Chalasia of the esophagus is a rare condition characterized by constant incompetence at the cardioesophageal sphincter [1]. Fluoroscopic examination shows that external pressure on the infant's barium-filled stomach always produces regurgitation of the contrast material into the esophagus, and that the cardiac sphincter remains wide open. Gravitational reflux is constant. True chalasia of the esophagus is rare. The radiologist should not confuse normal regurgitation with chalasia; the significance and incidence of varying degrees of chalasia are not clear.

Considerable controversy surrounds the incidence, identification, and significance of *hiatus hernia* in infants. The gastro-esophageal junction is best demonstrated with the infant in the prone left posterior oblique position, as an umbrella-shaped opening seen through the gas in the fundus of his stomach [2, 8]. The parallel, longitudinal folds of the esophagus meet the divergent gastric folds and form a readily identifiable "umbrella" (Fig. 9a). Movement of the cardia of the stomach above the diaphragm is common and may be normal. Eructation in the prone position is associated with a small transient hiatus hernia (Fig. 9a and b). This temporary hiatus hernia is the result and not the cause of *vomiting*. It must be differentiated from the pathologic condition in which a segment of stomach almost constantly lies above the diaphragm, the distal esophagus is irritable and may have an ulcer crater, and endoscopic examination shows signs of esophagitis. Hiatus hernias with peptic esophagitis are common in retarded infants and children who remain in the supine position for prolonged periods.

References

1. BERENBERG, W., NEUHAUSER, E. B. D.: Cardio-esophageal relaxation (chalasia) as a cause of vomiting in infants. Pediatrics **5**, 414 (1950)

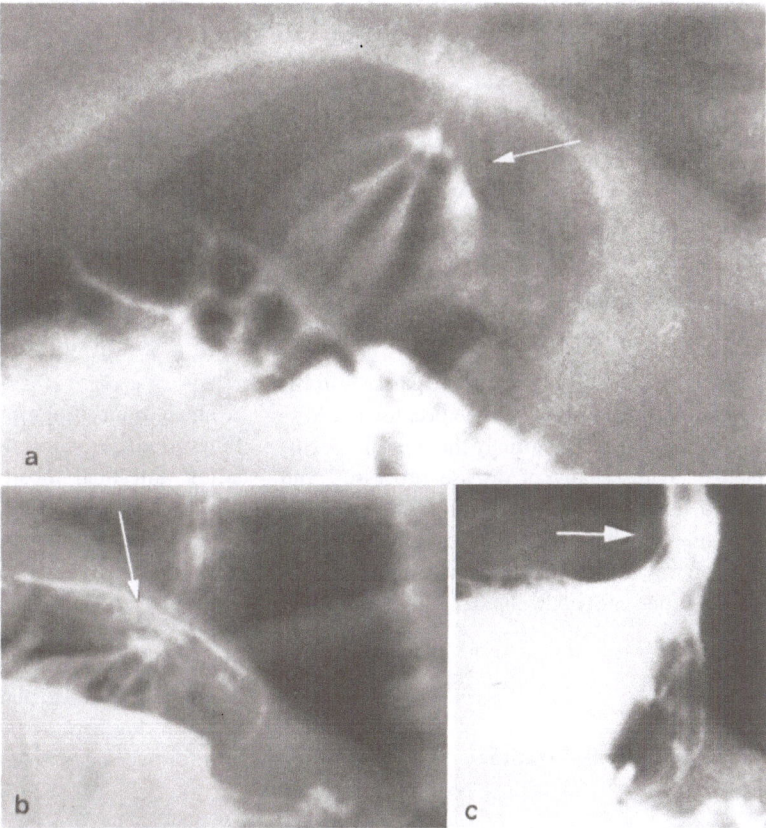

Fig. 9 a. Fluoroscopic spot film made with infant in prone oblique position shows normal gastroesophageal junction. Parallel folds of esophagus meet divergent gastric folds to form "umbrella" *(arrow)*. Air-filled fundus of stomach permits excellent visualization of cardioesophageal junction with the infant in this position

b) Normal esophageal junction

c) Small transient hiatus hernia in same infant during vomiting. Gastroesophageal junction was normal a few seconds later

From CAFFEY [2], with permission

2. CAFFEY, J.: Pediatric X-ray diagnosis, 6th ed. Chicago: Year Book Medical Publishers, Inc. Vol. I, pp. 580—607, 1972

3. CUMMINGS, W. A., REILLY, B. J.: Fatigue aspiration (a cause of recurrent pneumonia in infants). Radiology **105**, 387 (1972)

4. EKLÖF, O., LÖHR, G., OKMIAN, L.: Submucosal perforation of the esophagus in the neonate. Acta Radiol. (Diag.) **8**, 187 (1969)

5. GIRDANY, B. R.: The esophagus in infancy: congenital and acquired disease. Radiological Clinics of North America **1**, 557 (1963)

6. GIRDANY, B. R., SIEBER, W. K., OSMAN, M. Z.: Traumatic Pseudodiverticulum of the Pharynx in Newborn Infants. New Engl. J. Med. **280**, 237 (1969)

7. GWINN, J. L.: Tracheo-esophageal fistula with and without esophageal atresia—special aspects. Progress in Pediatric Radiology **2**, 170 (1969)

8. JUTRAS, A., LEVRIER, P., LONGTIN, M.: Etude radiologique de l'oesophage para-diaphragmatique et du cardia. Journal de radiologie et d'éléctrologie et archives d'éléctricitie medicale, Vol. 30, 373—414, 1949

9. MARGULIES, S. I., BRUNT, P. W., DONNER, M. W., SILBIGER, M. L.: Familial dysautonomia. Radiology **90**, 107 (1968)

10. OSMAN, M. Z., GIRDANY, B. R.: Traumatic pseudodiverticulums of the pharynx in infants and children. Annales de Radiologie **16**, 143 (1973)

11. SHEPARD, R., FENN, S., SIEBER, W. K.: Evaluation of the esophageal junction in postoperative esophageal atresia and tracheoesophageal fistula. Surgery **59**, 608 (1966)

Less Common Disease Patterns in the Gastro-Intestinal Tract with a Special Note on Meconium Ileus

R. Astley

1. Introduction

The subject of less common disease patterns in the alimentary tract has been chosen because it allows opportunity to mention briefly the typical appearances of a miscellany of disease processes, and then to point out just a few of the less typical forms that may be encountered, especially the less common ways in which relatively common conditions can present, both clinically and radiologically.

2. Oesophageal Atresia

This follows such a standard pattern that only simple X-ray procedures are required in most cases; it is debatable whether contrast studies are necessary as a pre-operative routine. A chest radiograph, with a radio-opaque tube passed to the point of obstruction, will show the occasional unusually low type of the anomaly as well as demonstrating the state of the lungs and whether or not gas has passed distally through an associated tracheo-oesophageal fistula.

Associated urogenital tract abnormalities in oesophagel atresia are uncommon. A recent review by my colleague John Lee showed that 10 out of 54 consecutive cases had urinary tract anomalies but 7 of these occurred in children who also had ano-rectal atresia; of the remaining 3, in only one was the lesion (pelvi-ureteric obstruction) likely to be significant, and this was not asymptomatic. Therefore it is suggested that routine urography in oesophageal atresia, unless it is complicated by ano-rectal atresia, is not a worthwhile procedure.

3. Isolated (H-type) Tracheo-oesophageal Fistula

A small tracheo-oesophageal-fistula may sometimes produce a clinical picture deceptively simulating intestinal obstruction, and pulmonary problems may be only a small part of the clinical picture. The radiological clues to plain film diagnosis in such babies are gaseous distension of both small and large bowel (and also, at times, the oesophagus) with gas extending distally all the way to the anus, the absence of horizontal fluid-levels and the co-existence of pulmonary changes with varying areas of consolidation and/or collapse or over-distension.

4. Achalasia

Achalasia is generally a condition of later childhood; it is extremely rare in babies and it is wise to be very suspicious of such a diagnosis in a young subject.

5. Chronic Granulomatous Disease

Oesophageal involvement in chronic granulomatous disease produces appearances somewhat like achalasia. Phagocytosis is normal in this condition but the ingested bacteria are not killed; indeed, they are protected within the polymorpho-nuclear cells from the action of antibiotics and continue to release toxic products. Intermittent or chronic infections with suppuration and granu-

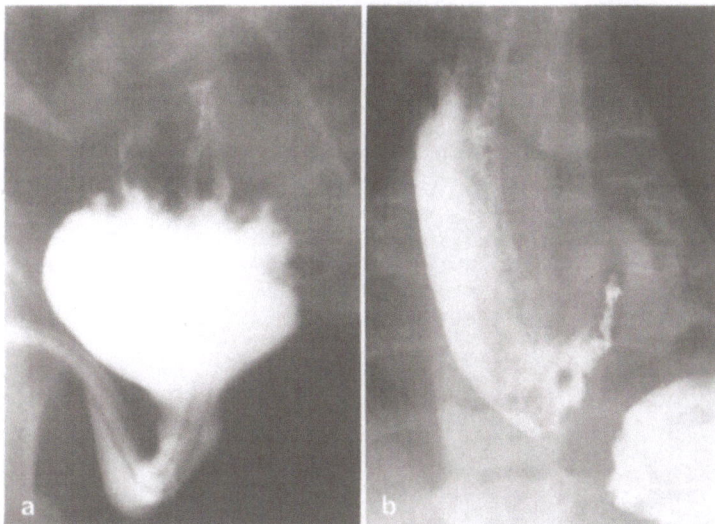

Fig. 1a and b. Chronic granulomatous disease. a) Filling defect due to involvement of bladder. Subsequent intravenous urography showed a normal upper tract but it was noted that lower thoracic paravertebral soft-tissues were widened. This led to a barium meal examination that showed asymptomatic oesophageal involvement. b) Oesophagus is wide and poorly contractile, with a surrounding soft-tissue mass

loma formation result. Males predominate, with symptoms usually beginning in early life, and ending in death before the adult state is reached. All parts of the body may be involved but the sites with radiological manifestations are most likely to be the *bones* (osteomyelitis, particularly in the small bones of the hands and feet, where it can sometimes resemble tuberculous dactylitis), *liver*, *urinary tract* (infection, ureteric obstruction by retroperitoneal fibrosis, involvement of the bladder), cardiovascular system (pericarditis, narrowings of major vessels, nonspecific cardiomegaly) and *lungs*. There are protracted pulmonary infections with hilar adenitis and massive or patchy consolidation that is slowly revolving and leaves linear opacities. There may be bronchiectasis, lung abscess or empyema.

Oesophageal involvement by mediastinitis is frequent but often asymptomatic. Sutcliffe and Chrispin [13] found oesophageal abnormalities in four out of eight patients. The oesophagus is widened slightly or considerably and shows poor emptying movements (Fig. 1b). There is oesophageal stasis when lying down, decreasing in the erect position; hiatal function is good, with no reflux and no evidence of oesophagitis. There is usually a thickened band of soft tissues along the oesophageal border and often a soft-tissue mass around it, particularly extending to the left behind the heart. A sinus may lead from the oesophagus into the mass.

6. Hiatal Hernia

In childhood, a hiatal hernia usually produces a suggestive history. The vomiting varies in character from regurgitant to frankly projectile but it almost always commences within the first few days of life and in over 90% the vomitus at some time contains blood, although usually only as a few brown streaks. Similarly, the radiological picture is often very definite, with identification of a small loculus of stomach above the diaphragm associated with *abnormal* gastro-oesophageal reflux.

The word "abnormal" must be emphasized; reflux in a baby is not necessarily abnormal, particularly if there is much gaseous distension and the tests for gastro-oesophageal incompetence are severe.

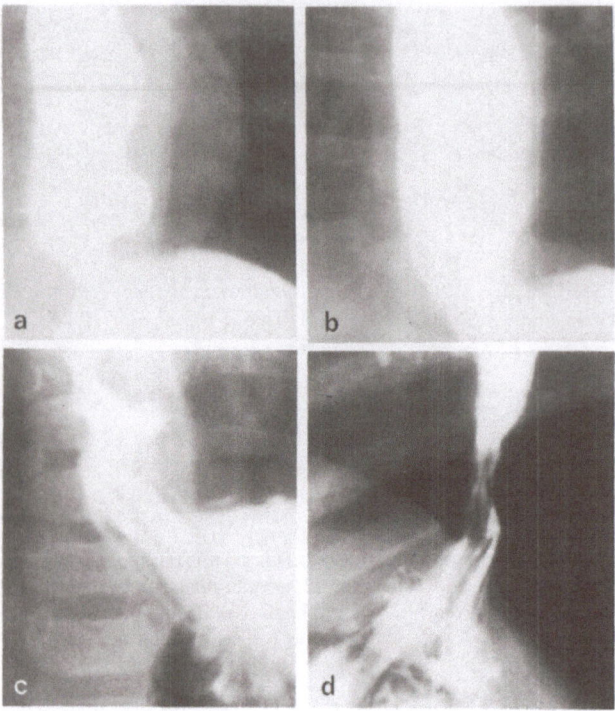

Fig. 2. Hiatal hernia simulating "chalasia". Male, age 4 months. Four spot films taken during the same examination. In the upper two, a mistaken diagnosis of "chalasia" would be possible; demonstration of the mucosal pattern shows a small hiatal hernia

Demonstration of the anatomical abnormality is usually a safer ground than assessment of the ease of producing reflux.

Radiological mistakes occur in both directions. Over-diagnosis results if the criteria for identifying the herniated stomach in the chest are not strict enough. Under-diagnosis occurs mainly for two reasons. Firstly, it must be realised that sometimes the abnormality may reveal itself very fleetingly and therefore its possible presence must be very much in the observer's mind during careful fluoroscopy. Manual pressure on the abdomen below the xiphoid while the baby is swallowing barium suspension, to ensure adequate distension of the lower part of the oesophagus, is an essential part of the procedure and so is study of the mucosal pattern. Secondly, the small hiatal hernia may be missed if we believe that the condition of so-called chalasia exists as anything but a rarity (Fig. 2).

Atypical clinical presentation of a small hiatal hernia can occur in various ways. The presenting feature is occasionally anaemia. Oesophageal bleeding with a small hernia is mostly evident in the early weeks of life but massive haemorrhage is rare. Later on, it is often not a feature unless peptic ulceration with a reflux stricture of the oesophagus develops (it is estimated that this happens in about 5% of cases). Very occasionally, however, even in children without a stricture, there may be sufficient blood loss, as repeated small melaenas, to produce a significant anaemia. Beyond infancy, vomiting due to a hiatal hernia may be a relatively unimportant feature in the history, and its role may not be realised in the production of the anaemia.

Chest infections in hiatal hernia are occasionally the main clinical feature; these are probably similar in their causation to those seen in achalasia, and related to a small over-spill of regurgitated food into the tracheo-bronchial tree, probably occurring during sleep. Any child with recurrent or persistent chest infections needs a contrast study of the oesophagus, not only to exclude hiatal hernia but also any other possible cause of aspiration such as disordered swallowing or a small isolated tracheo-oesophageal fistula.

Simulation of oesophageal atresia by a hiatal hernia can occur in the first few hours of life, with cyanotic attacks and frothy fluid at the mouth. Radiologically, there is disturbance of swallowing produced by the transmission of intra-abdominal pressures into the oesophagus. It may be necessary to re-examine a few days later (when the incoordination of swallowing will usually be less) to demonstrate the hiatal hernia.

Spastic obstruction at the lower end of the oesophagus due to oesophagitis associated with a small hiatal hernia produces another atypical radiological presentation in the newborn. Here again repeat examination after a few days, when the spasm has abated under treatment, may be necessary to show the hernia; it must be remembered that oesophagitis can occur due to vomiting that is not associated with a hernia.

Other developmental anomalis that may be associated with hiatal hernia include the interesting group of conditions that may be grouped under the broad heading of *duplications of the foregut*, including thoracic, gastric, enteric and bronchogenic cysts, pulmonary cysts and sequestrated lobes. These anomalies occur in various combinations and with a variety of other associated features such as malrotation of the midgut and anomalous blood supply direct from the aorta. Of 11 cases [1], 5 had a small hiatal hernia. The association of foregut duplications with a bifid cervical or thoracic vertebral body or narrowed disc space is a well-known diagnostic clue.

The microgastria syndrome usually includes a hiatal hernia. The thoracic loculus of stomach runs into the remainder of the stomach in a midline position (Fig. 3). The stomach is small, vertical in position and often tubular in shape, with its pylorus directed downwards. Anomalous midgut rotation may be shown by absence of the duodenal loop and a right-sided position of the small intestine. Other malformations are common: asplenia (with Howell-Jolly bodies in the blood); transverse position of the liver; congenital heart disease, most commonly an endocardial cushion defect; abnormal pulmonary lobulation; intestinal obstruction (e.g. oesophageal atresia, duodenal atresia, imperforate anus). One of the two cases

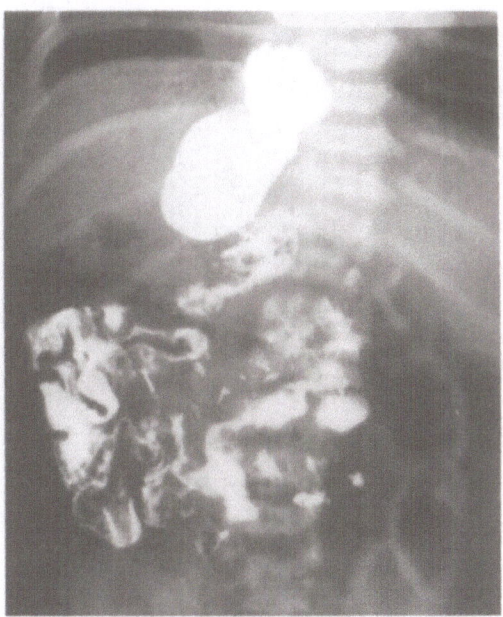

Fig. 3. Micro-gastria. The small stomach is almost vertical, with part of the fundus above the diaphragm. There is no duodenal loop and the upper jejunum lies on the right, indicating anomalous rotation of midgut

described by SHACKELFORD et al. [11] had HIRCHSPRUNG's disease of the whole colon and SCHULZ's case [10] had skeletal anomalies.

7. Hypertrophic Pyloric Stenosis

Later presentation, at 2 to 5 months of age instead of at the classical 2 to 3 weeks after birth, is an occasional variant of the clinical picture.

Gastric pneumatosis, the gas within the wall of the stomach producing a halo of translucency, is a rare complication of pyloric stenosis that does not necessarily imply a poor prognosis (Fig. 4).

8. Peptic Ulceration

The increase in the incidence of peptic ulceration in childhood may be partly due to the wider realisation that the clinical history in this age group is

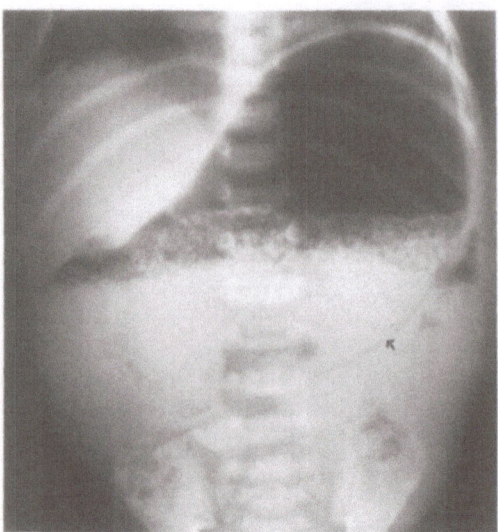

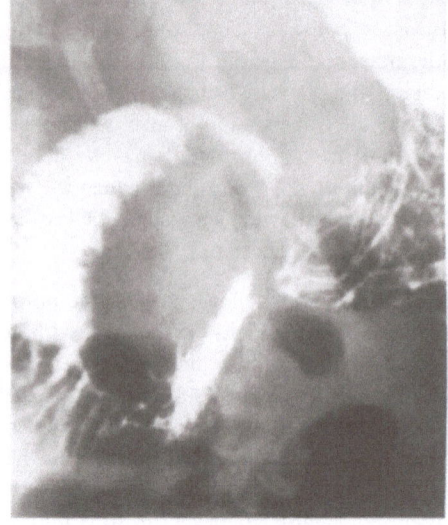

Fig. 4. Gastric pneumatosis in hypertrophic pyloric stenosis. Note the thin "halo" of gas in the wall of the distended stomach *(arrow)*. Normal response to pyloromyotomy

Fig. 5. Pancreatitis. Female, age 10 years. Acute abdominal pain and vomiting. Slightly widened duodenal loop with "rounded appearance", coarse mucosal folds and slightly slowed transit. Raised serum amylase level

Table 1. Presenting features in 40 children with peptic ulceration

Pain (± tenderness) 32	
	Not a feature in 8
	Mild in 3
	Related to food in 13
	Related to excercise 2
Vomiting 21	
Haematemesis and/or melaena 13	

apt to be less typical than in the adult (Table 1). In particular, the relationship to food may be poorly defined. Fortunately the radiological appearances are more typical than the clinical features.

9. Acute Pancreatitis

Like peptic ulceration, this is more frequently recognized in childhood once its existence is remembered. There is a considerable number of possible causes but two-thirds fall into the idiopathic group (MUSTARD et al. [8]). There is usually no associated biliary tract disease. When there is a known cause, it is usually trauma—blunt abdominal injuries, occasionally direct injury at surgery (e.g. during splenectomy). Roundworms in the pancreatic duct may be important in countries where these parasites are common. Mumps pancreatitis is rare or mild in childhood. Steroids, used therapeutically, provide another occasional cause.

The majority present with intermittent abdominal pain or as an acute surgical abdomen (HENDREN et al. [2]). The preoperative diagnosis is apt to be acute appendicitis or peritonitis. However, if the possibility of pancreatitis is considered, the serum amylase level and radiology can give help (Fig. 5).

SLOVIS et al. [12] drew attention to the association of pancreatitis with nonaccidental injuries (the battered-child syndrome). In one abused child that they described, traumatic pancreatitis was associated with bone changes due to fat necrosis; in another it was associated with multiple fractures and the authors emphasize the need to have both possibilities in mind. While the bone changes secondary to pancreatitis include periosteal change, they are predominantly lytic, with destructive lesions that are not seen with fractures.

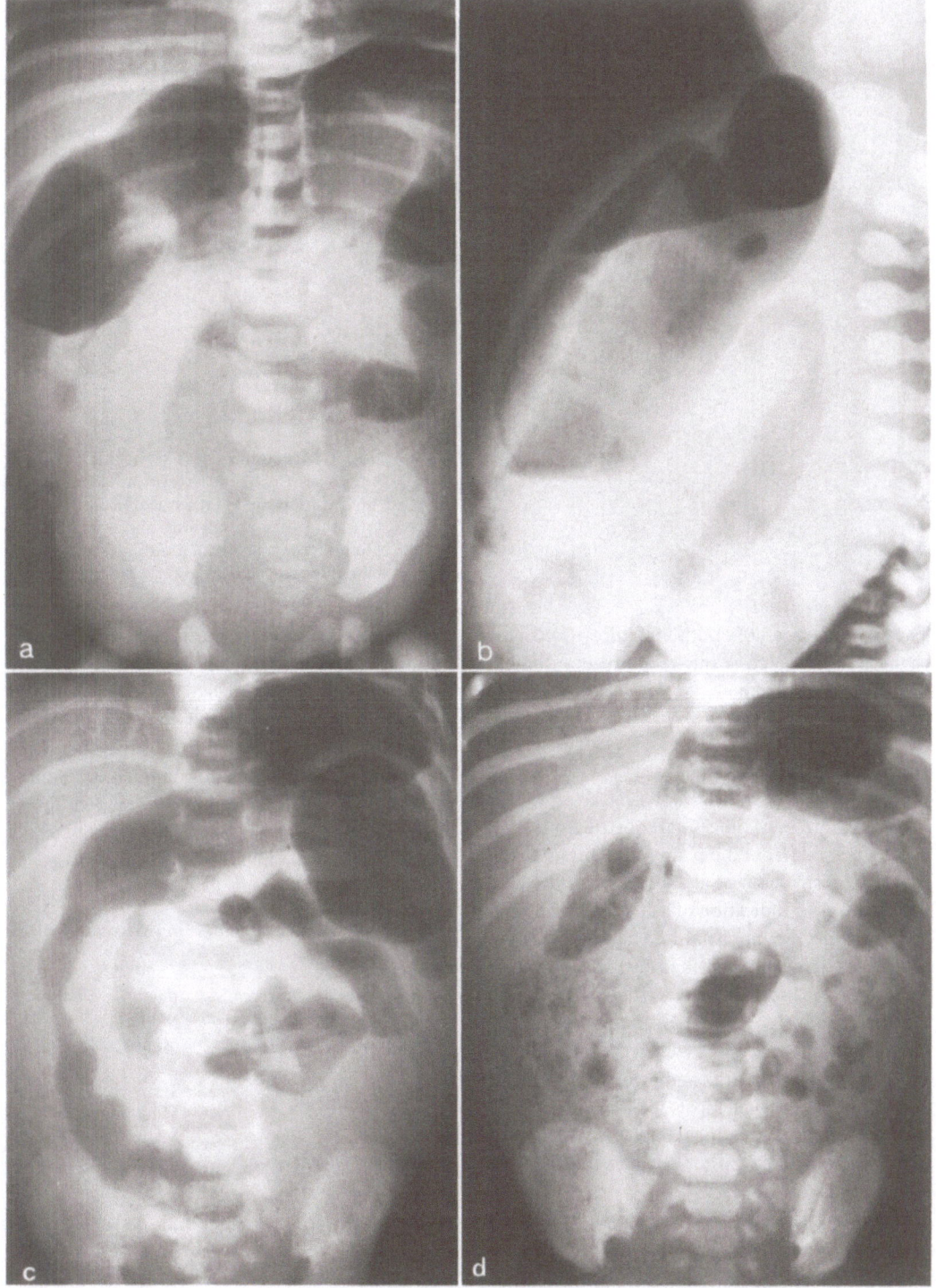

Fig. 6 a—d. Meconium ileus; typical findings. a) Erect and b) lateral inverted views. Very distended but not very numerous loops of small bowel; scanty fluid levels; meconium mottling; varying calibre or tapering loops (note loop like a "rolled umbrella" in lateral view!); no gas in the rectum. c) Erect. A good example of varying calibre of loops; scanty fluid-levels; a little meconium mottling in right flank. d) Erect. Much meconium mottling of a coarser type than often seen; not many distended loops; scanty fluid-levels

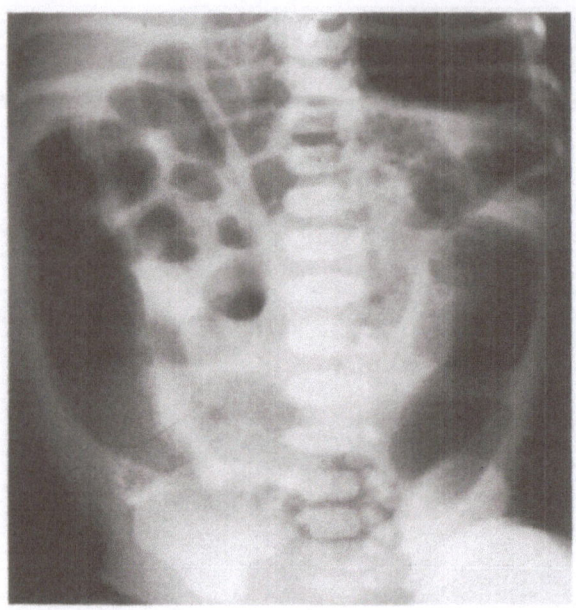

Fig. 7. Meconium ileus; slightly less typical findings. Erect. The greater number of distended loops makes it more difficult to recognise that they are all small intestine. Scanty fluid-levels; meconium mottling; slight tapering of loops (see right lower quadrant)

The co-existence of both fractures and the changes of fat necrosis might produce a difficult medico-legal problem.

10. Meconium Ileus

In many forms of intestinal obstruction it is usually possible from the plain radiographs to decide that obstruction is likely to exist, but there may be no clear indication of its cause. Meconium ileus provides an important exception; KALAY-OGLU et al. [5] estimated that in this condition a correct diagnosis of the cause of the obstruction can be made in 65% while HOLSCLAW et al. [4] put the figure at nearly 75% when the radiological and clinical evidence are combined. This possibility of pre-operative diagnosis is fortunate in view of the conservative treatment, especially by hypertonic water-soluble contrast enemas, that is often used nowadays.

The radiological signs are those of intestinal obstruction with a triad of additional signs (Fig. 6).

The obstruction shows itself by gaseous distention of small bowel but the colon is usually empty of all but traces of gas. Fortunately, in meconium ileus, although some loops may be very large indeed, the number of distended loops is often not great, so that it is often fairly easy to recognise that there are gas-free regions and to decide that these "empty" areas are likely to represent the colon. In some, however, there are multiple distended loops that occupy much of the abdomen, presenting the problem that is frequent in infancy, i.e., deciding whether multiple distended loops represent small intestine plus colon or only small bowel (Fig. 7). This may be impossible to decide

Table 2. Plain film findings in Meconium Ileus (37 cases)

Dilated loops	Few	8
	Moderate	18
	Many	11
Very large loops		15
Fluid-levels	Scanty	25
	Moderate	9
	Many	3
Varying loop calibre	+ +	13
	+	15
	O	9
Meconium mottling	+ + +	4
	+ +	20
	+	13
	O	0
Rectal gas	O	75
	Trace	6
	+ +	2
	?	4

Table 3. Radiological signs in 37 cases of meconium ileus

Case No	Signs Favouring M.I.			Against M.I.		
	Meconium mottling	Varying calibre	Scanty levels	Multiple levels	Rectal[a] gas	Diagnostic difficulty
5	□ □ □	□	□			
23	□ □ □	□ □	□			
3	□ □ □	□ □	□			
8	□ □ □	□ □	□			
2	□ □ □	□ □	□			
7	□ □	□ □	□			
9	□ □	□ □	□			
12	□ □	□ □	□			
26	□ □	□ □	□			
36	□ □	□ □	□			
6	□ □	□ □				
10	□ □	□ □				
24	□ □	□				
14	□ □	□				
4	□ □	□	□			
17	□ □	□	□		■ ■	■ ■
16	□ □	□	□			
33	□ □	□	□			
13	□ □		□			
27	□ □		□			
15	□ □					
11	□ □					
25	□ □			■ ■ ■		
1	□ □	·		■ ■ ■	■ ■	■ ■
35	□	□ □	□			
37	□	□ □	□			
34	□	□	□			
31	□	□	□			
32	□	□	□			
22	□		□			
20	□		□			■ ■
19	□		□			■ ■
28	□		□			■ ■
29	□	□				■ ■
18	□					■ ■
21	□					
30	□			■ ■ ■		■ ■

In each column, number of squares indicates assessment as + + +, + + or +.
The last column on the right indicates the cases where in actual practice there was difficulty in making the diagnosis from the plain films.
[a] More than a trace of gas in the rectum.

without a contrast enema. The tubular form of the loops and their size often do not allow distinction between small and large intestine. Identification of gas in the rectosigmoid as it turns towards the anus is often the most certain guide. A lateral inverted picture is invaluable in this respect; if there is gas in the distal colon it rises into the pelvis, towards the anus. In meconium ileus the inverted lateral picture will usually show no gas or only a few spots in the recto-sigmoid.

The first of the triad of additional features is really a negative one; horizontal fluid-levels are apt to be scanty or absent because of the sticky nature of the contents of the gut in cystic fibrosis.

The second additional feature is the presence of meconium mottling, varying from a fine, ground-glass appearance to a coarser variety. HERSON [3] found meconium mottling in two-thirds of cases and KALAYOGLU et al. in about a half.

The third member of the triad is the presence of varying calibre in one or several of the small intestinal loops, which taper from one width to another. This is a manifestation of the "string of sausages" appearance that the small bowel presents at operation or necropsy.

Table 2 shows an analysis of the plain film findings in 37 cases of meconium ileus, excluding those presenting with meconium peritonitis. It is seen that the dilated loops were few or moderate in number in about 70%, with varying calibre in 75% and scanty fluid-levels in 68%. Some amount of meconium mottling was present in all cases and was graded as + + or + + + in 65%. Rectal gas was more than a trace in only 2 cases. In Table 3 these findings are set out in another way and it is seen that a combination of signs favouring meconium ileus was present to a vary-

ing degree in the majority of cases; multiple levels and/or more than a trace of rectal gas were present in only 4 cases and in practice there was diagnostic uncertainty (as far as plain film diagnosis was concerned) in 8 cases out of 37 (22%). This is an agreement with the previously mentioned figures of 65–75% for plain film diagnosis.

In any assessment of the value of radiological signs, we must consider *false positives* as well as false negatives. *It must be emphasised that none of the signs of meconium ileus is completely specific* (Figs. 8, 9). LEONIDAS et al. [6] found only 25% of uncomplicated cases with no fluid-levels, but they agreed that very prominent fluid-levels were unusual. Thus, the scantiness is a relative matter. As they pointed out, it can be produced falsely if intestinal suction has removed much of the accumulated fluid above a simple atresia. Conversely, there are some cases of meconium ileus that *do* have multiple fluid-levels. LEONIDAS thought that their presence suggested a complication such as an atresia, but we have seen them on occasion in uncomplicated meconium ileus and they were not

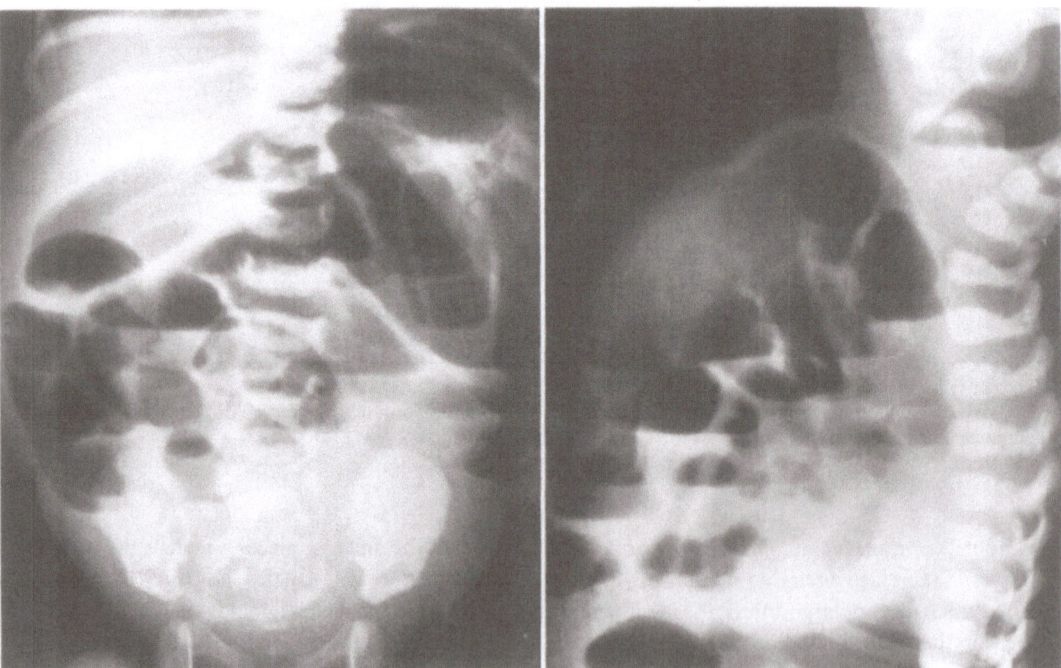

Fig. 8. Meconium ileus; atypical findings. Erect and lateral inverted views. Multiple very distended loops with many fluid-levels; some meconium mottling; much gas and a fluid-level in the rectum

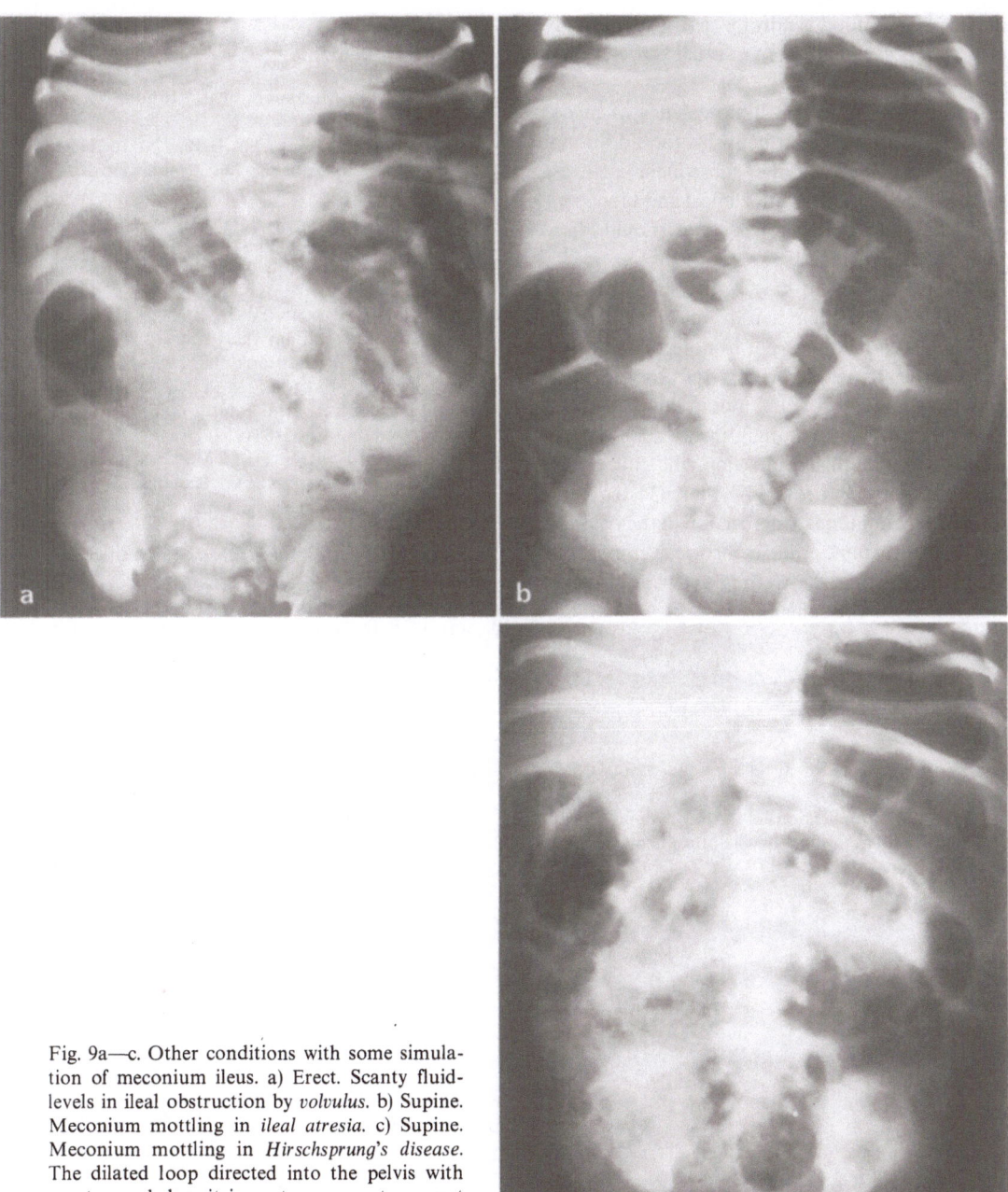

Fig. 9a—c. Other conditions with some simulation of meconium ileus. a) Erect. Scanty fluid-levels in ileal obstruction by *volvulus*. b) Supine. Meconium mottling in *ileal atresia*. c) Supine. Meconium mottling in *Hirschsprung's disease*. The dilated loop directed into the pelvis with scanty gas below it in rectum suggests correct diagnosis

present in the complicated cases in the present series. Indeed, detection of complications seems to be very difficult.

Meconium mottling is also a nonspecific sign that is seen in a variety of conditions. In all of these it is not necessarily situated in the small bowel but it may not be possible to make this distinction. It can be seen in colonic obstructions such as HIRSCHSPRUNG's disease, imperforate anus, temporary meconium obstruction of the newborn and the inspissated food syndrome. Most confusingly of all, it is occasionally seen in small bowel atresia without meconium ileus.

In addition to the plain film evidence of meconium ileus, there will usually be the additional findings provided by the subsequent contrast enema; these, together with clinical and biochemical findings and the child's progress should allow a correct diagnosis.

It is not proposed to discuss the subject of the treatment of meconium ileus by enemas of hypertonic contrast media except to note that the medium originally used for this purpose, Gastrografin [9], is no more efficacious in our experience than other iodine-containing media such as Hypaque 25%. In this connection, the finding by LUTZGER and FACTOR [7] that Gastrografin causes more inflammatory reaction in the colon of rats than do some other nemedea is important. They suggest that the wetting agent additive in Gastrografin is the damaging factor.

References

1. ASTLEY, R.: Duplications of the foregut and related conditions. Acta chir. belg. Supplement II, 79—159 (1960)

2. HENDREN, W. H., GREEP, J. M., PATTON, A. S.: Pancreatitis in childhood. Arch. Dis. Childh. **40**, 132—145 (1965)

3. HERSON, R. E.: Meconium ileus. Radiology. **68**, 568—571 (1957)

4. HOLSCLAW, D. S., ECKSTEIN, H. B., NIXON, H. H.: Meconium ileus. Amer. J. Dis. Child. **109**, 101—113 (1965)

5. KALAYOGLU, M., SIEBER, W. K., RODNAN, J. B., KIESEWETTER, W. B.: Meconium ileus: a critical review of treatment and eventual progress. J. pediat. Surg. **6**, 290—300 (1971)

6. LEONIDAS, J. C., BERDON, W. E., BAKER, D. H., SANTULLI, T. V.: Meconium ileus and its complications. Amer. J. Roentgenol. **108**, 598—609 (1970)

7. LUTZGER, L. G., FACTOR, S. M.: Effects of some water-soluble contrast media on the colonic mucosa. Radiology **118**, 545—548 (1969)

8. MUSTARD, W. T., RAVITCH, M. M., SNYDER, W. H., WELCH, K. J., BENSON, C. D.: Pediatric Surgery. Second Edition. Page 751. Chicago: Year Book Publishers 1969

9. NOBLETT, H. R.: Treatment of uncomplicated meconium ileus by Gastrografin enema; a preliminary report. J. pediat. Surg. **4**, 190—197 (1969)

10. SCHULZ, R. D.: Microgastrie congénitale. Ann. Radiol. **14**, 285—287 (1971)

11. SHACKELFORD, G. D., MCALISTER, W. H., BRODEUR, A. E., RAGSDALE, E. F.: Congenital microgastria. Amer. J. Roentgenol. **118**, 72—76 (1973)

12. SLOVIS, T. L., BERDON, W. E., HALLER, J. O., BAKER, D. H., ROSEN, L.: Pancreatitis and the battered child syndrome. Amer. J. Roentgenol. **125**, 456—461 (1975)

13. SUTCLIFFE, J., CHRISPIN, A. R.: Chronic granulomatous disease. Brit. J. Radiol. **43**, 110—118 (1970)

Small Intestine — the Terminal Illeum Loop

M. A. Lassrich

Radiological examination of the small intestine in children has to be very carefully considered because of the radiation exposure which accompanies such studies. Even so, radiological study of the small intestine is often necessary and the reason is that quite a large number of acute and chronic abdominal and intestinal diseases, important clinical syndromes and distinctive symptoms, are all especially amenable to radiological assessment. For example, radiological studies can be helpful in certain acute abdominal diseases, regurgitation and continuous vomiting, chronic diarrhoea or steatorrhea, abdominal distension or protracted fever of unknown origin. Radiological examination of the small bowel is important when there is bleeding which cannot be localised to the oesophagus, stomach, duodenum or colon. In addition, in patients with abdominal tumours or severe or recurrent pain, radiological examination can be helpful. Naturally this list is not complete, but it sets out in a broad and general way the reasons why radiological studies can provide the decisive information which leads to rational clinical management.

In recent years there has been renewed interest in the small bowel and an awareness that many diseases which involve this segment of the alimentary system can be diagnosed quite accurately by careful attention to their radiological features. Several factors have stimulated progress. These include new perspectives of the pathology of the small intestine, information from endoscopy and biopsy, improvements in the techniques of radiological examination, and, last but not least, better radiological equipment, such as image intensifiers, television video-tape record systems, new low dose intensifying screens and fluorographs. Nowadays the radiation dose is considerably lessened [4, 6–8, 14, 15] by comparison with former times.

In small intestinal examinations we pay more attention to anatomical alterations than to functional disturbances. The detection of anatomic lesions is more diagnostic and, therefore, clinically more relevant. Functional disturbances which are observed often symbolize evidence of the second rank only.

For verifying anatomical lesions the so-called "fractional filling" method has yielded the best results. We use the following technique: After the examination of the stomach and duodenum has been completed, the child is put to lie on his right side in a horizontal position. When more contrast medium is given he remains in this position. Then—sip by sip—the child is fed an additional 100 to 150 ml of contrast medium (1 to 2 sips every five minutes). With this technique of feeding, the stomach fills the small intestine in a physiological way. About 20 to 30 minutes after starting the procedure, the upper two thirds of the small intestine is opacified. The time taken differs from child to child and the study must be controlled fluoroscopically. As soon as the contrast medium reaches the lower ileum a radiograph is taken with the child in the prone position. In the normal child the small intestine is seen as a continuous shadow which presents a uniform and harmonious aspect. This standardized technique also provides a certain amount of information about alterations in function.

To detect anatomical lesions it is absolutely essential to check every intestinal loop. This is possible only during episodes of fluoroscopy when adjacent loops can be separated by the palpating hand of the radiologist. Palpation has to be carried out very gently and carefully in order not to evoke resistance: nevertheless, it must be systematic so that no region of the small intestine is not studied. Only with this method of examination can ana-

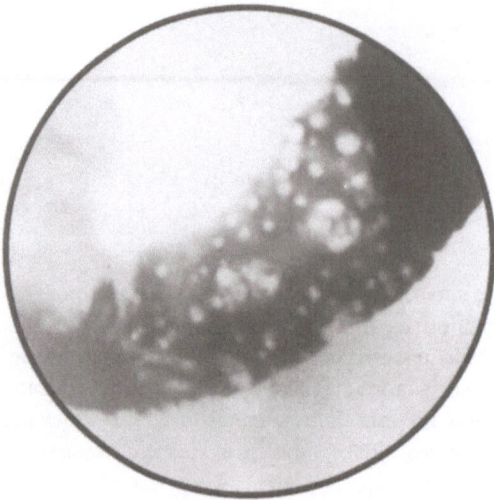

Fig. 1. Spot film of an ileal loop in a 12 year old child. Study during convalescence after a small bowel infection. Polypoid filling defects of different size, corresponding to isolated enlarged lymph follicles and Peyer's patches

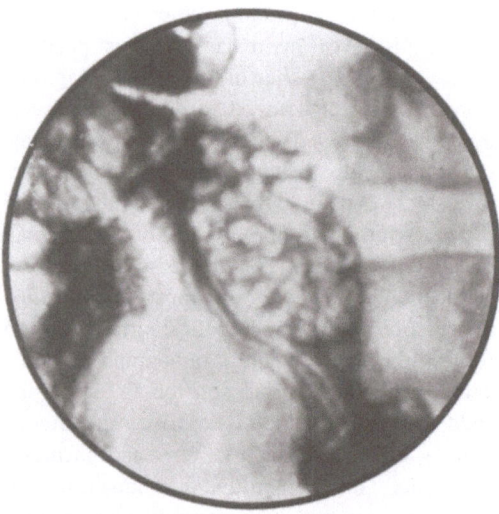

Fig. 2. Spot film of the terminal ileum in a 7 year old child. Large sized Peyer's patch: at its base is a polypoid structure, caused by enlarged lymph follicles

tomical details be identified with certainty and recorded. A technique of examination which is restricted solely to radiographs is not adequate for it will not yield all the information required for clinical decisions.

The timing of fluoroscopy study is determined by the speed of transit of contrast medium. The size of the fluoroscopic field is always limited to a small area. A large area cannot be observed precisely, and, furthermore, it increases radiation dose. Pathological findings detected during fluoroscopy are recorded on spot films which must be made with appropriate compression. Only in this way is it possible to demonstrate minor but important pathological changes, and to record them without confusing interference from superimposed loops. Pathological changes or anatomical variants need to be verified with certainty with a second spot film and maybe a repeated filling procedure.

Difficulties may occur during examination of the lower ileum. The convolutions of superimposed loops may be hard to differentiate and separate by palpation for they lie huddled together in the child's small pelvis.

The terminal ileum and the ileo-caecal region are always easy to demonstrate by using this technique. However, it must be pointed out that the contrast enema has also proved to be suitable for examination of the lowermost ileal loops when reflux of barium into the small intestine can be achieved. This is usually possible in children. Whichever method is used to study the distal ileum only a sensible combination of fluoroscopy and radiography will give consistently good diagnostic results.

A wide range of diseases of the small intestine may be studied radiologically, but only a few of these will be discussed. Conditions affecting the lower small intestine, especially the terminal ileum, are emphasized in particular. Changes in the mucous membrane, the intestinal wall and the regional lymph nodes are considered.

In children we normally find well developed lymphatic tissue in the mucosal and submucosal layer of the small bowel and especially in the terminal ileum. This tissue lies in a multiplicity of lymph follicles and Peyer's patches. In the distal ileum well developed but normal lymphatic tissue produces a characteristic X-ray appearance. A polypoid mucosal change, with nodular protrusion is a characteristic of lymphatic tissue hyperplasia. When, for example, this tissue is inflamed the radiographic appearances change.

From pathological specimens we have obtained a general idea about the amount of the lymphatic tissue in the small intestine. But long-standing and emaciating disease produces a considerable reduction in the whole of the lymphatic tissue. Therefore, it is often not possible to transfer an experience based on pathological specimens to the normal living child. However, we have seen that in children who have died suddenly there is always very well developed lymphatic tissue and this corresponds with the normal situation.

In radiographs of the distal ileum of 130 apparently healthy children aged between 2 and 14 years, we found an age-dependent pattern. The lymph follicles develop variably and their size corresponds to the age of the child. The peak of lymph follicle development lies within the age range 4–9 years. Additional factors which influence this development are the status of the alimentary tract and the kind of food the child eats. Later on, as puberty approaches and general involution of the lymphatic tissue takes place, the lymph follicles in the mucosal layer of the small bowel also diminish in number and size. During

this time we can see a changing pattern in the distal ileum tending towards that found in adults, as time passes. This is why we observe in older children a mucosal pattern devoid of polypoid changes [5, 11, 20].

Certain reactive changes can be observed and demonstrated with spot films. Such changes in the lymphatic tissue we can see regularly during and after infections affecting the GI tract.

In addition some of the typical infectious diseases of childhood (such as scarlet fever, tonsillitis, infectious mononucleosis, measles or German measles etc.), involve the entire lymphatic tissue of the body including that in the small bowel. Clinically we can sometimes note pain in form of "pseudoappendicitis" or similar discomforts. Naturally, these children do not always need an X-ray examination, but sometimes other diseases or appendicitis need to be excluded.

Regularly, we can observe a reactive enlargement of lymph follicles in the distal ileal loop after reduction of an acute intussusception. We consider

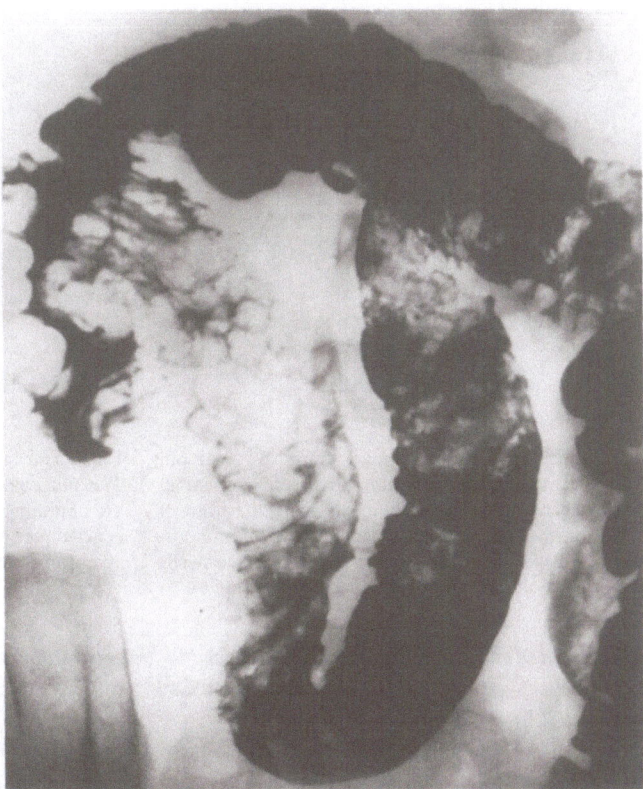

Fig. 3. 10 month old infant. Radiograph of the ileocaecal region after reduction of an acute intussusception. Oedema of the caecal pole and the ileocaecal valve shown with enlarged lymph follicles in the distal ileum

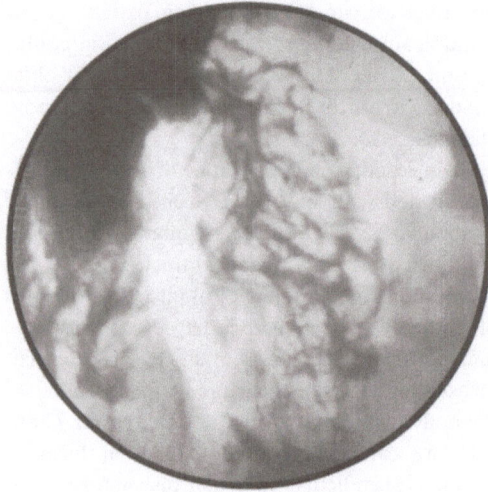

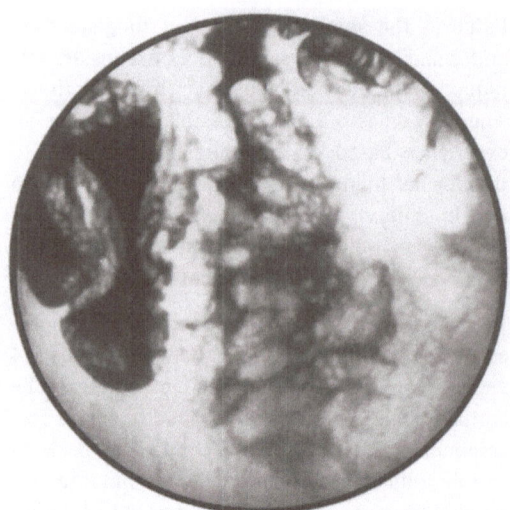

Fig. 4. Spot film of the terminal ileum in a 12 year old child with scarlet fever, complaining of abdominal pain in the right lower quadrant of the abdomen, enlargement of the lymph follicles. Normal findings 4 weeks later

Fig. 6. 10 year old child with nonsclerosing ileitis (Golden). Spot film of the terminal ileum. Patchy filling defects resulting from marked enlargement of the lymph follicles and Peyer's patches. The thickened loop could be palpated and was sensitive to pressure

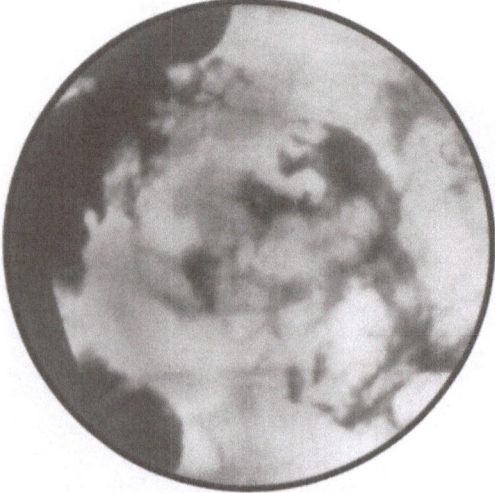

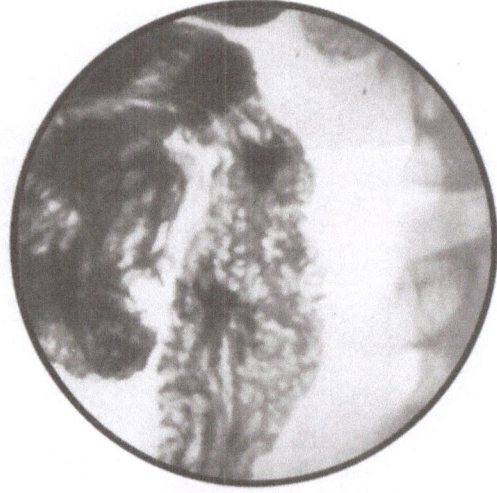

Fig. 5. Spot film of the terminal ileum in a 5 year old child with measles. Examination during the prodromal phase. Severe abdominal pain in the right quadrant of the abdomen. Enormous enlargement of the lymph follicles and Peyer's patches as a feature of reactive swelling of the whole lymphatic tissue

Fig. 7. The same child as in Figure 6, 10 months later. The mucosal relief has become normal—the follicles are of almost normal size. The terminal loop of ileum is no longer palpable or sensitive to pressure. Clinical symptoms and abdominal pain no longer present

the reactive changes of lymphatic tissue, especially of the Peyer's patches, as *one* factor which can lead to an intussusception.

In cases of nonsclerosing ileitis (Golden) we have been able to analyze the acute changes and ob-serve their course. These children complain about rather non-specific pain in the right lower quadrant of the abdomen or abdominal colic which may sometimes simulate appendicitis. In the radiograph and during fluoroscopy, we can observe

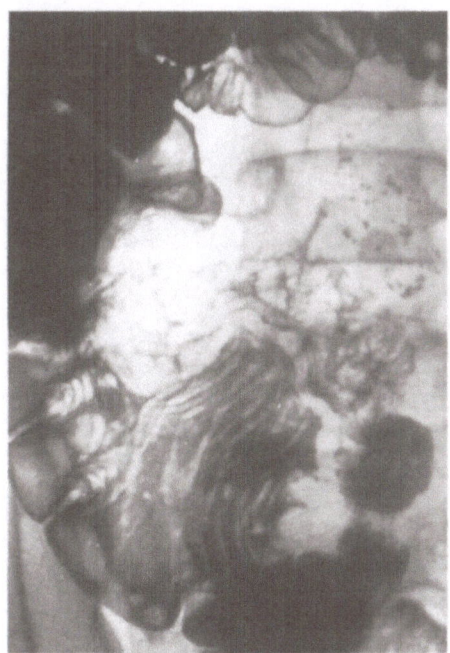

Fig. 8. Tumefaction of the ileocaecal valve in nonsclerosing ileitis. Marked oedema of both lips narrows the outlet of the terminal ileum and the valve protrudes into the caecal lumen. Lesion palpable and tender

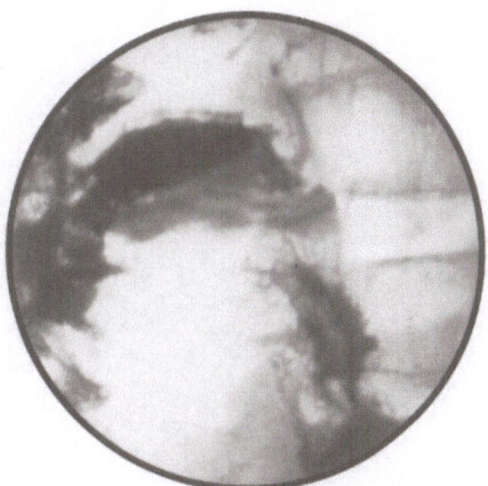

Fig. 9. 6 year old tuberculin-positive child with primary intestinal tuberculosis. No fever, no diarrhoea. Only the spot film of the terminal ileum showed the extensive mucosal changes with ulceration of the enlarged lymph follicles and Peyer's patches. The contours are eroded and the normal pattern of mucosal folds and follicles is absent

in the terminal ileum those patchy filling defects which are caused by marked enlargement of the lymph follicles and Peyer's patches. Clinically, the thickened wall can be felt as a sausage-shape, its position can be localised at fluoroscopy, and, when palpated it is painful. Contractility of the affected segment is diminished and there may also be swelling of the ileocaecal valve, and enlarged ileocaecal lymph nodes. In some cases these radiological findings were verified during laparotomy. We consider that various harmful factors can produce either chronic or acute inflammatory processes in the terminal loop of the ileum: these ileal changes parallel the pathological conditions in infections which are so frequently observed in the pharyngeal lymphatic tissue [1, 3, 10, 16, 18].

In tuberculous infection of the small bowel (primary tuberculosis) the point of entry of the organism is almost always obscure. Furthermore, in most developed countries tuberculosis nowadays represents neither a diagnostic nor a therapeutic problem. Nevertheless, the mode of infection and

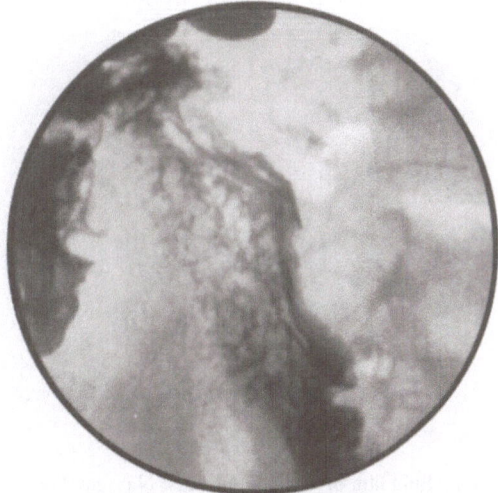

Fig. 10. The same child as in Figure 9, but two years later. In the previously ulcerated region there is now flat scar formation. Return to a normal mucosal and follicular pattern is evident. Incipient calcification of the ileocaecal lymph nodes

the corresponding small bowel reaction, together with characteristic radiographic findings are very important as a model for other types of bowel infection and bowel reaction.

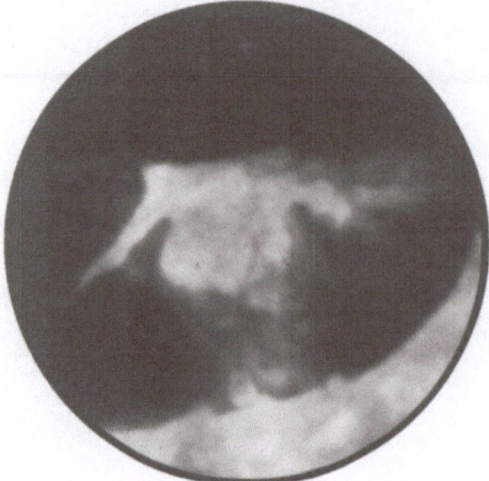

Fig. 11. Spot film of the terminal ileum in a case of typhoid fever in a 9 year old child in second week of illness. Enormous enlargement of the follicles and Peyer's patches affected by this specific inflammatory process

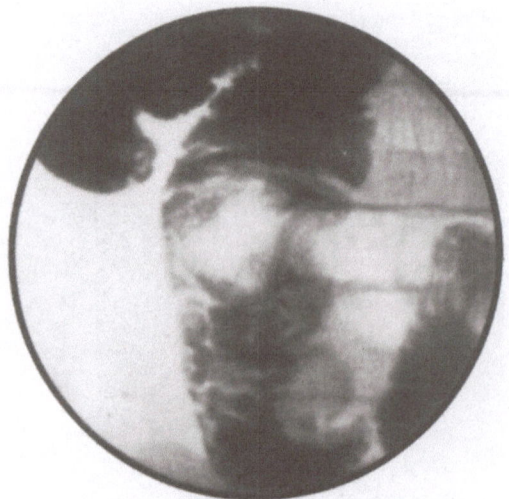

Fig. 13. 11 year old child. Spot film of terminal ileum with a circumscribed filling defect, caused by an enlarged non-calcified lymph node, demonstrated with controlled compression

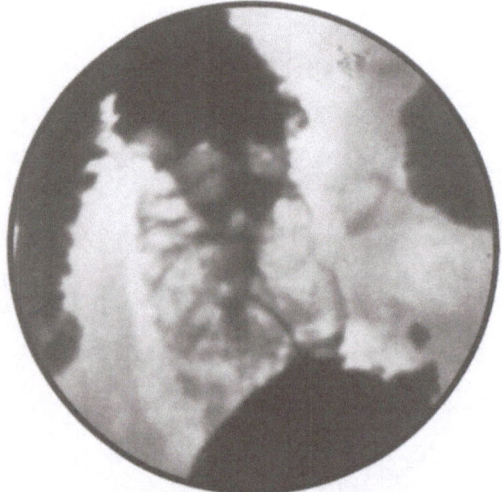

Fig. 12. Spot film of the ileum in a case of typhoid fever. Large filling defects with narrowing of the lumen, due to swollen and enlarged Peyer's patches

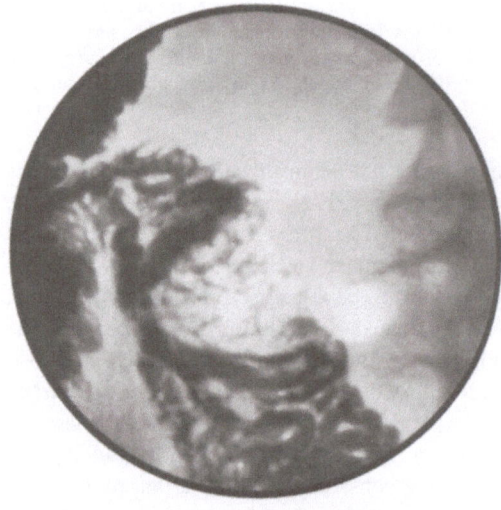

Fig. 14. Spot film taken with controlled compression, demonstrating a non-calcified lymph node near an ileal loop

The primary mucosal lesion becomes localised in the lymph follicles and Peyer's patches and there is a concomitant reactive enlargement of the mesenteric lymph nodes. In most cases the point of entry of the tubercle bacillus disappears and there is no local cicatrization at that site. But the infected Peyer's patches can ulcerate superficially.

Later on a plateau-like mural filling defect, corresponding with an enlarged Peyer's patch may, develop. Symmetrical or asymmetrical annular narrowing of an ileal loop can occur as scar tissue forms [2, 17].
In typhoid fever similar radiographic findings can be observed and it may be almost impossible to

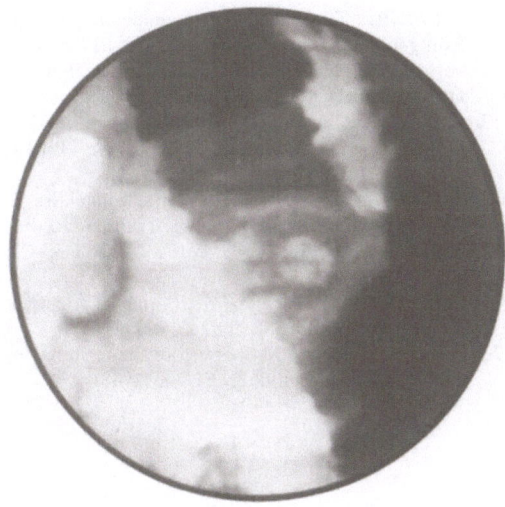

Fig. 15. Solitary well defined polyp in a 5 year old child with periumbilical colic. The polyp could only be identified after careful palpation and separation of the different loops

tinal loops themselves. On the other hand, small or only moderately large tumours of the mesentery (e.g. small aggregates of lymph nodes or individual nodes) require special attention and an appropriate technique of examination. The local pressure effect of the small mass becomes evident when the individual small intestinal loops are pushed apart and compressed against enlarged lymph nodes, for it is not possible to smooth out the profiles of the loops by palpation during fluoroscopy. When the pressure of palpation is released these filling defects disappear, but they can be reproduced by renewing the pressure. These phenomena are observed in non-specific and specific diseases of the mesenteric lymph nodes. Such a finding is clinically important in cases of tuberculosis, when, for example, there is only slight evidence of calcification, or maybe no calcification at all, or when there needs to be certainty as to whether the lymph nodes are affected or not [4, 9].

differentiate these from those of tuberculosis. Clinical information and additional data are obviously necessary. In typhoid fever the changes are best seen in the lower ileum, where the lymph follicles may show remarkable swelling and the Peyer's patches are enlarged. The swollen patches give the impression of a tumour-like formation, surrounding and narrowing the bowel lumen. In both diseases, tuberculosis and typhoid fever, there are also non-specific features with nothing that can be regarded as characteristic of either tuberculosis or typhoid fever: these include patchy filling defects, hypersecretion, acceleration of transit time, segmentation, and alterations in tone. Only spot films reveal typical changes and are essential for diagnosis.

Enlargement of the mesenteric lymph nodes is common in children and we can find such nodes in nearly all infections of the small bowel. Furthermore, they occur in a great number of other diseases. A diagnosis of mesenteric lymph node enlargement by clinical observation, examination or palpation is not possible. However, enlargement of any structure contiguous with the small bowel may cause displacement and compression of small intestinal loops. In this way large tumours tend to produce displacement of the intes-

References

1. ARNULF, G., BUFFARD, P.: L'iléite lymphoide terminale. Presse méd. **61**, 107 (1953)
2. BÖHM, F.: Untersuchungen über die Tuberkulose des Dünndarms. Stuttgart: Georg Thieme 1950
3. BÜCKER, J., FEINDT, H. R.: Pseudopolyposis lymphatica ilei (Pseudoileitis). Fortschr. Röntgenstr. **74**, 59 (1951)
4. BUFFARD, P.: Étude radiologique des adénopathies iléo-caecales de l'enfant. Pédiatrie **40**, 877 (1951)
5. CHÉRIGIÉ, E., DEPORTE, A., TAVERNIER, C., MME PRADEL-RAYNAL: Le grêle terminal de l'enfant. Étude anatomique, anatomo-pathologique et radiologique. Ann. Radiol. **5—6**, 319 (1959)
6. CHRISPIN, A. R.: Radiological examination of the small intestine in children. In: Progress in Pediatric Radiology, Vol. **2**, 211. Basel/Year Book, Chicago: Karger 1969
7. GOLDEN, R.: Radiologic examination of the small intestine. Philadelphia-London-Montreal: J. B. Lippincott Co 1945
8. KIRSNER, J. B., SHORTER, R. G.: Inflammatory bowel disease. Philadelphia: Lea & Febiger 1975
9. LASSRICH, M. A.: Röntgendiagnostik unverkalkter abdomineller Lymphknoten beim Kinde. Z. Kinderheilk. **73**, 319 (1953)
10. LASSRICH, M. A.: Die nichtsklerosierende Ileitis beim Kinde. Z. Kinderheilk. **74**, 50 (1953)

11. LASSRICH, M. A.: Röntgenologische Studien an der terminalen Ileumschlinge bei gesunden Kindern. Z. Kinderheilk. **74**, 77 (1953)

12. MARINA-FIOL, C., R. CARBALLO: Exploración del ileon terminal. Rev. clin. esp. **3**, 97 (1941)

13. MARINA-FIOL, C.: El diagnostico de la tuberculosis intestinal en su comienzo. Revista clin. esp. **11**, 81 (1943)

14. MARSHAK, R. H., LINDNER, A. E.: Radiology of the small intestine. Philadelphia-London-Toronto: W. B. Saunders Company 1970

15. PORCHER, P., BUFFARD, P., SAUVEGRAIN, J.: Radiologie clinique de l'intestine grêle de l'adulte et de l'enfant. Paris: Masson & Cie. 1954

16. PRÉVÔT, R.: Die nichtsklerosierende Ileitis. In: Röntgendiagnostik, Ergebnisse 1952—1956, herausgeg. von H. R. SCHINZ, R. GLAUNER, E. UEHLINGER. Stuttgart: Georg Thieme 1957

17. PRÉVÔT, R.: Röntgendiagnostik der Darmtuberkulose. In: Handbuch der Tuberkulose, Bd. IV, S. 601. Stuttgart: Georg Thieme 1963

18. SAUVEGRAIN, J., NAHUM, H.: Iléite folliculaire et adénolymphite mésentérique. In: Traite de Radiodiagnostic, Vol. **18**, p. 215. Paris: Masson & Cie 1973

19. STRÖMBECK, J. P.: Terminal ileitis and its roentgen picture. Acta radiol. (Stockh.) **22**, 827 (1941)

20. WELLS, J.: The mucosal pattern of the terminal ileum in children. Radiology **51**, 305 (1948)

Current Views on the Diagnosis of Colonic Aganglionosis

B. J. Cremin, V. Boston, and D. Brockwell

1. Introduction

The contributions of FREDERICK RUYSCH [25] and HARALD HIRSCHSPRUNG [18] in describing congenital megacolon are well documented.

It took 60 years after the first clear clinical presentation and description before the deficiency of the nervous plexuses in the distal narrow segment of the large bowel was generally accepted [28]. This quickly led to the animal research laboratory where ORVAR SWENSON developed his pull-through procedure.

Today, surgical manipulation remains empirical, because knowledge of the basic sciences of anatomy, physiology and pathology is incomplete. One of Nature's more subtle experiments continues to defy exact definition, and though many are now salvaged, much suffering is still endured.

The affected bowel is considered to be normal except for its nerve supply. By definition, in Hirschsprung's disease the innervation of the smooth muscle of the internal anal sphincter is always abnormal, and this extends for a variable distance proximally. However, the traditional concepts of pre- and postganglionic autonomic fibres are no longer considered valid. In giving a brief description of current concepts, an attempt will be made to give the reasons for the distribution of the intramural plexus abnormality and the disparity between the size of the distal abnormally innervated bowel and the dilated transitional zone.

2. Pathogenesis

The theory of the embryogenesis of the intramural intrinsic nervous system given by OKAMOTO and UEDA [24] in their classical contribution found a cranio-caudal migration of foetal neuroblasts from the cranio-cervical neural crest region to the anus. These neuroblasts mature and migrate lumenward through the circular muscle layer to form the inter-myenteric (AUERBACH'S), the submucosal (MEISSNER'S), and then eventually the mucosal plexus. The bundles of the extrinsic fibres (parasympathetic and sympathetic) ramify before sinking into the wall of the gut to synapse with the various plexuses. The postulate pertaining to the embryogenesis of Hirschsprung's disease states that there is an arrest of this initial craniocaudal migration of neuroblasts. As the internal anal sphincter is the last and most distal structure to be innervated by these migrating neuroblasts, it must always be affected in Hirschsprung's disease. The length of the "aganglionosis" therefore depends at what state this migratory arrest occurs.

3. Pathophysiology

There are several controversial hypotheses concerning the disparity of gut lumen in aganglionosis. There are three abnormal zones present in the alimentary tract in Hirschsprung's disease. In the distal narrow zone the intrinsic component of the intramural plexus is absent. This is considered to be composed of three functional groups of fibres which are 1. motor effector—argyrophobic, cholinergic (which inhibit excitation-contraction coupling in smooth muscle [8, 29]); 2. co-ordinating internuncial—argyrophilic, cholinergic [27]; and 3. a separate motor effector system—argyrophobic, purinergic (which has adenosine triphosphate as its transmitter substance) [5], which is responsible for the phase of distal receptive inhibition of smooth muscle during normal peristalsis. It should be clearly understood that the extrinsic adrenergic and cholinergic nerve supply and the underlying nuncial environment can only modify quantitatively the function of this intrinsic component of the intramural plexus.

The observed rhythmical electrical activity of gut smooth muscle is thought to be activated by a spontaneous myogenic source, which causes myogenic contraction. The function of the cholinergic argyrophobic fibres is to inhibit the activity of this spontaneous source. It follows that any stimulation by these intrinsic nerves can only result in myogenic inhibition. Without this inhibitory mechanism a hypertonic state exists.

The loss of the internuncial communicating neurones results in the disappearance of progressive coordinated reflex peristaltic activity.

Loss of the purinergic nerves in the affected segment in Hirschsprung's disease results in failure of distal receptive relaxation following proximal distention.

Another factor contributing to the "narrowed" calibre of the distal segment may be the direct effects of excessive acetyl choline produced by the hypertrophic infiltrating preganglionic sacral parasympathetic fibres acting on smooth muscle. Other possibilities may be Cannon's hypothesis of denervation hypersensitivity [6], and the abnormal distribution of stimulating adrenergic receptors creating an abnormal segment that behaves like a long internal anal sphincter [1]. These mechanisms interacting in an unplanned manner cause the functional obstruction, and this results in the proximal dilatation. Poor propulsive activity resulting from the inadequate innervation present in the transitional zone compounds this effect.

4. Diagnosis of Hirschsprung's Disease

A reliable diagnosis of Hirschsprung's disease can be achieved in the majority of cases, but occasionally it is equivocal, and in these circumstances the accumulated evidence from many sources may improve diagnostic efficiency. Clinical, radiological, manometric and histological parameters will therefore be reviewed in this communication, with emphasis on points which are recognised to give rise to confusion in interpretation.

4.1. Clinical Diagnosis

The classic description of the child with Hirschsprung's disease presenting with severe constipation, a distended abdomen, wasted limbs and stunted growth has become a rarity in most parts of the world as a majority of cases are now diagnosed in early infancy. During the 20-year period 1957–1976, 214 cases of congenital intestinal aganglionosis were referred to the Red Cross Children's Hospital, Cape Town, of which 171 (80%) were the short segment variety (involvement as far as the rectosigmoid colon), 27 (13%) were long segment and 16 (7%) total colonic aganglionosis. The short segment variety had the usual 3:1 male to female sex ratio while the total colonic cases had an equal sex incidence (7 male, 9 female). None of these cases was premature, and in the latter 10 years of this period [10], 90% of the cases were in the neonatal period. Most patients presented with intestinal obstruction within a few days of birth. In the less acutely affected children, attacks of intermittent and sometimes explosive diarrhoea alternated with constipation, and these symptoms dated from birth.

Necrotising enterocolitis associated with the disease represented a diagnostic dilemma. Differentiation from a primary septicaemia with secondary paralytic ileus frequently proved difficult, the more so because of the urgency of surgical treatment.

4.2. Radiological Diagnosis

Radiological diagnosis of this condition in the neonate is not always easy [2, 9, 14, 19]. The difficulties are discussed from the point of view of a) the abdominal survey radiograph, b) the barium enema, and c) the delayed radiograph.

a) All our cases presented with some degree of obstruction and showed variable degrees of dilated bowel or fluid levels on the survey film. If early diagnosis is to be made there should be a high degree of suspicion for this condition on all cases of intestinal obstruction, particularly when other causes such as atresia and meconium ileus have been eliminated.

We obtain an inverted lateral radiograph in all our cases of neonatal intestinal obstruction. It is

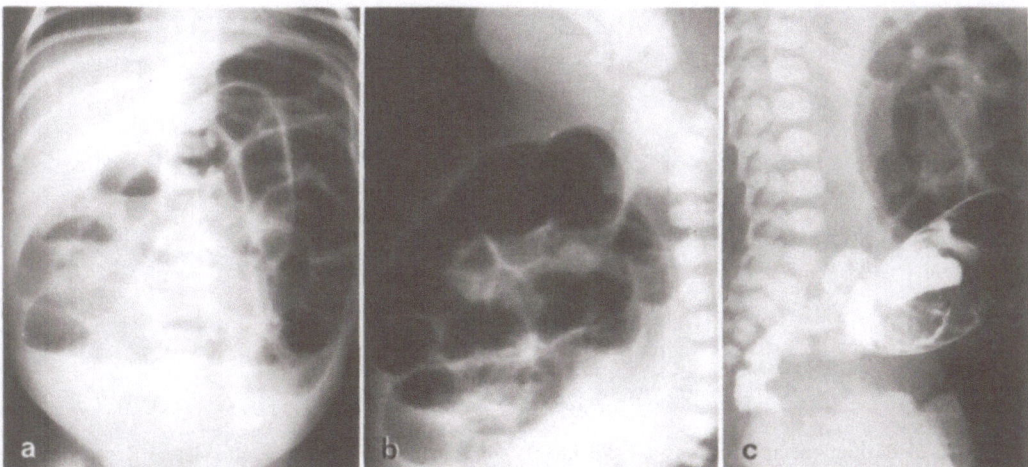

Fig. 1 a–c. a) Frontal erect radiograph showing multiple fluid levels
b) Inverted lateral radiograph demonstrating distension of gut and lack of gas in rectal area. This feature suggests Hirschsprung's disease

c) Same case (3-day-old male). In view of plain radiograph findings a careful enema was performed and this demonstrates a fairly well marked transition zone in the "early" delayed film

our routine practise, and no hazards have been encountered. Although the value of this radiograph has not gained widespread radiological acceptance it enables an objective assessment of fluid levels from a lateral dimension and an estimate of gaseous distension of the lower bowel. All cases that show either a complete or relative absence of rectal gas in the inverted lateral film are particularly suspected of having Hirschsprung's disease, and a meticulous barium enema study is made in these cases (Fig. 1). In geographical areas where gastroenteritis is prevalent as a cause of infantile paralytic ileus, the inverted film will be more likely to show a rectum fully distended with gas on the inverted film and rule out Hirschsprung's disease as a cause of obstruction.
b) The major difficulty in barium enema diagnosis is that a clear-cut narrowed "aganglionic" transition zone is not always evident and may not be visible during the filling stage of the examination. An established narrow zone usually takes a week or two to develop [14] and can easily be obscured during the examination. The appearances can be variable, and relatively common are either a coned or more gradual tapering of a tunnel-funnel type of transition zone; this is the one in which most radiological mistakes are made (Figs. 2, 3).

Techniques of examination vary even amongst experienced paediatric radiologists, but our preference is to use a simple small rubber catheter and a hand syringe injection of 30% wt/vol solution of

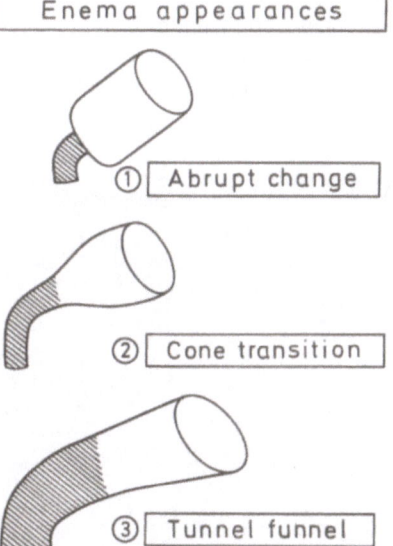

Fig. 2. An abrupt change in transition zone is not the commonest appearance in neonates, more common is a longer coned transition. A gradual "tunnel funnel" appearance is not uncommon and can make diagnosis difficult, particularly in filling stage

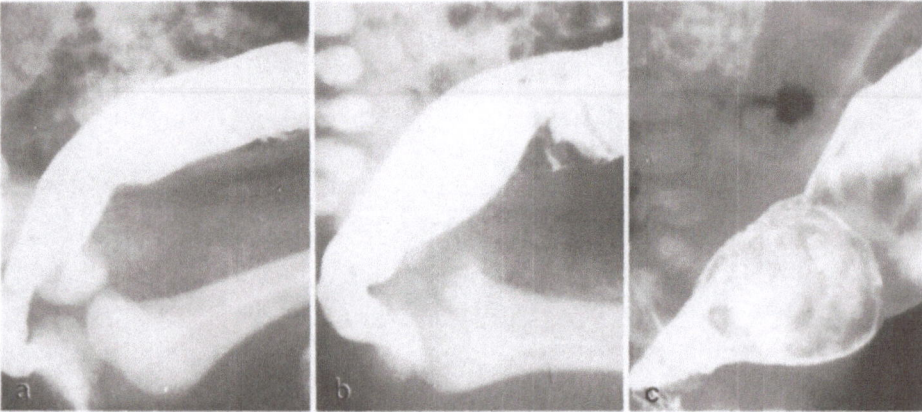

Fig. 3a–c. a) Barium enema in a four-day-old infant showing "tunnel funnel" appearance with a lack of appreciable change in transition zone
b) "Early" delayed film. Appearances were not recognised as aganglionosis and the radiographic error was compounded by not ordering a "late" delayed film

c) Same case. Three months later. Repeat barium enema shows the abrupt changes diagnostic of Hirschsprung's disease

barium sulphate. The infant is unprepared and preliminary wash-outs are contraindicated as they are liable to distort the subsequent radiological appearances. We have had no incidence of water intoxication in the neonatal age group. This condition is more likely to arise in the older child who has been over-enthusiastically washed out and given a large enema. To retain the catheter, many radiologists use adhesive strapping, but our preference is for manual compression of the buttocks.

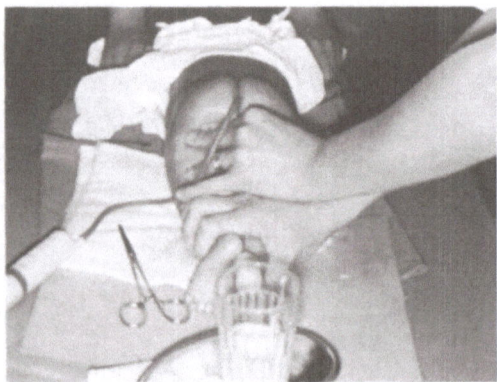

Fig. 4. Baby in prone position at start of barium enema. Left thumb and forefinger squeeze buttocks and right hand restrains legs (they are collimated out of direct X-rays and further protected from the undercouch tube by placing a lead sheet on table and under hands)

The compression is done by thumb and forefinger and the X-ray beam collimated so that the digits are not exposed to radiation. This is more easily performed by commencing the examination in the prone position and turning to the lateral position once the rectosigmoid is filled (Fig. 4). At this stage we stop injecting barium and wait a few minutes so that the effects of distention are diminished before radiographs are taken. The use of manual compression to prevent the leakage of barium will not be universally condoned and requires experience in the technique if radiation to the hands is to be avoided. We have monitored the hand in this technique and recorded no appreciable effects after three minutes of fluoroscopy [10]. As our table is equipped with an undercouch tube we take the additional precaution of placing a sheet of lead rubber on the table and under the restraining hand. We prefer not to use any form of self-retaining catheters as this may result in overfilling; inflatable balloon catheters are dangerous at this age, particularly in the hands of the uninitiated.

The radiologist should use a technique with which he is familiar, but in neonates this should include the basic essentials: 1. avoidance of overdistension and overfilling, 2. careful observation of the rectosigmoid in oblique and lateral positions and 3. no haste in taking radiographs. We take a radiograph just after the catheter has been removed and before the patient is taken off the table. This we call the "early" delayed radiograph (Fig. 5).

c) The "late" delayed radiograph is taken 12–24 h after the examination. It is performed in the lateral position to show a transition zone and retained barium. This radiograph can be extremely useful and is also our routine, except in cases when a complicating enterocolitis makes early surgery mandatory. In these cases waiting for a "delayed" late radiograph may be dangerous and misleading, because evacuation of barium is likely to occur with the accompanying diarrhoea.

Meconium plugs can mask the appearance of Hirschsprung's disease and as they are not infrequently associated with the condition, aganglionosis must always be excluded. When they are diagnosed, our present policy is to assist evacuation by completing the enema with Gastrografin (meglumine diatrizoate). Before this is done we note if the infant is sufficiently well hydrated, and the possible necessity of subsequent intravenous therapy. Transient motility disorders such as the recently described small left colon syndrome [12] should not present diagnostic difficulty as the transition zone is at the splenic flexure and is not a persistent feature in subsequent enemas. Many of the infants also have diabetic mothers.

Aganglionosis involving the whole colon differs from the short segment variety, epidemiologically, anatomically and functionally. The term Hirschsprung's disease, which implies a megacolon, can hardly be used to describe the condition. It may present variable features [11, 13, 16], ranging from some diffuse narrowing to apparent normality.
In a recent series of six cases [11] a spastic, irregular appearance that simulated enterocolitis was not infrequently present, but the major diagnostic feature was unprovoked reflux into a narrow terminal ileum that showed a proximal megaileum (Fig. 6). Overfilling in these cases is cautioned against as proximal reflux may be extensive [7].

Our experience of delayed radiographs in this condition has been in cases referred from other hospitals in which there has been complete retention of barium lasting for days after the examination was performed (Fig. 7). Any case which has, on plain radiographs, small intestinal obstruction,

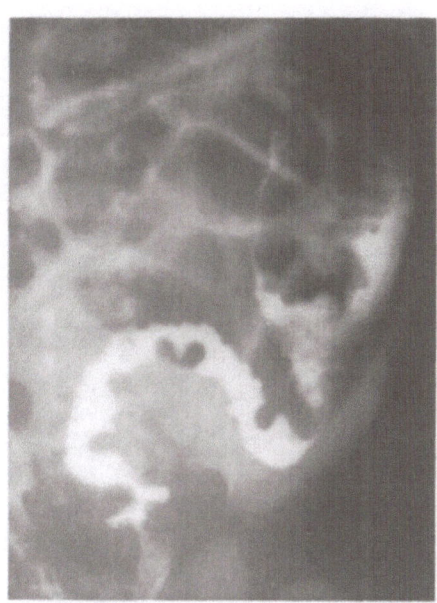

Fig. 5. "Early" delayed film demonstrating narrowed aganglionic colon and well-marked cone transition zone

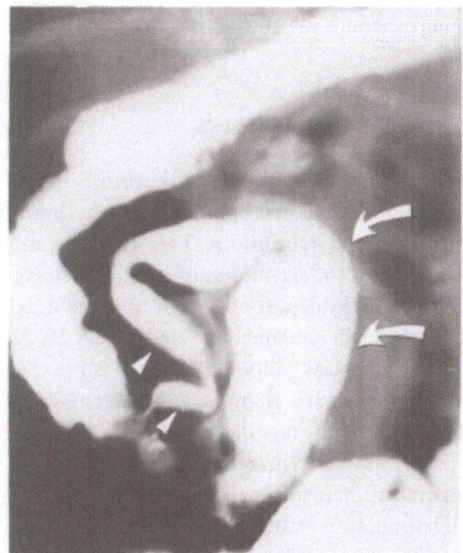

Fig. 6. Total colonic aganglionosis with reflux into narrow aganglionotic terminal-ileum *(arrowheads)* and dilated proximal mega-ileum *(curved arrows)*

no remarkable features in the colon apart from spastic irregularity, but has unprovoked ileal reflux with a distended ileum should be suspected, and a laparotomy with multiple frozen section biopsies performed.

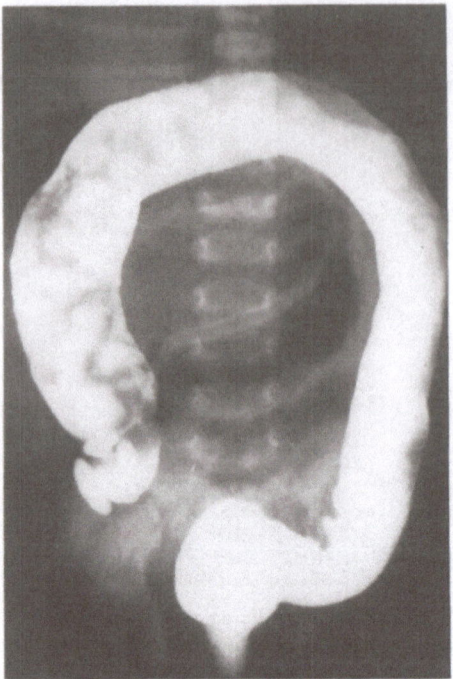

Fig. 7. Total colonic aganglionosis showing complete retention of barium, four days after initial examination

4.3. Manometric Diagnosis

In basic terms, when the normal rectum is distended the internal anal sphincter will be inhibited (this implies relaxation). This reflex is mediated through the intramural plexus. In Hirschsprung's disease this will not occur and the internal sphincter will remain contracted [3, 17, 20, 21, 26]. Using a special balloon catheter it is possible to monitor pressure changes in the anal canal while distending the rectum (Fig. 8).

The problems in interpretation are related to:
a) Identification of internal sphincter activity.
b) Determination of an appropriate rectal stimulus.
c) Movement artifact.

The pressure monitor in the anal canal does not solely measure the smooth muscle of the internal sphincter activity. Nett anal canal tone is the sum of activities of the internal sphincter and the striated muscle of the external sphincter and pelvic diaphragm. No problems would exist if the reflex activity of both groups were the same. However, this is not the case. The striated muscle

group, whose activity is mediated through a spinal reflex, first contracts with smaller, and then relaxes with much larger stimuli when the defaecation reflex is initiated.

b) Determination of internal sphincter activity
In general, an appropriate stimulus can only be determined by trial and error and this is usually one which is just less than that required to be appreciated at a conscious level, and thus it is possible to avoid precipitation of the defaecation reflex [3].

c) Movement artifact
Any movement of the subject during investigation will make interpretation impossible. It can be avoided by having the patient lie quite still and relaxed, preferably sleeping. This is particularly relevant in the neonatal period, where the pressure changes of interest are small relative to those created by movement. Much patience is usually required in achieving satisfactory observation conditions.

Diagnostic reliability can be in excess of 90% in optimal conditions [3, 20, 21].

4.4. Histological Diagnosis

The accepted definition of Hirschsprung's disease depends on the inability to identify ganglion cells in the affected segment of gut [28]. The intramural plexus is also abnormal in that the fibres are increased in size and number and there is infiltration of submucosa and mucosa with nerve fibrils [22]. Using histochemical stains these fibres are seen to be the source of increased concentration of the degrading enzymes of neuro transmitter substances. Meier–Ruge developed a histochemical staining method for acetylcholinesterase which aids identification of cholinergic fibres and ganglion cells [22]. Most centres in addition still use H & E staining methods on paraffin sections.

It must be remembered that the terminal approximately 1 cm of the alimentary tract normally has a decreased ganglion cell population and increased size and number of fibres [22]. Biopsies taken from this area should therefore be interpreted with caution. Age-dependent morphological changes in ganglion cells may also lead to confusion [4].

Full thickness biopsy is no longer fashionable; it requires a general anaesthetic and can make sub-

Measurement anorectal reflex

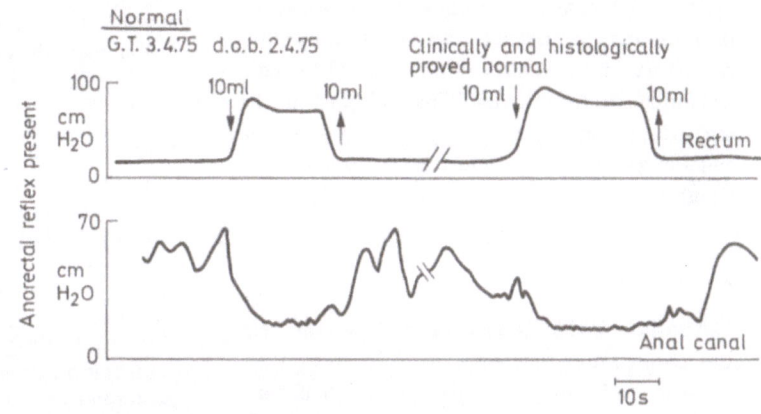

Fig. 8 a–c. a) A silicon rubber balloon has been placed in rectum at least 2 cm proximal to monitoring device in anal canal. A perfusion catheter utilising a constant fluid pressure enables internal sphincter activity to be assessed

b) Normal case showing anal sphincter inhibition (relaxation) on distending the rectum

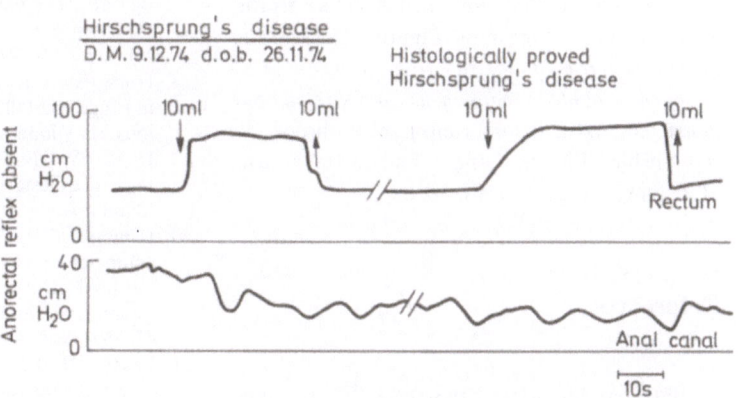

c) Hirschsprung's disease. No internal anal sphincter inhibition on rectal distention

sequent surgery more difficult. Suction biopsies (which contain muscularis mucosa) provide sufficient material for multiple-level sectioning, and examination [23]. With experience, providing adequate biopsy material is available, histological diagnosis will be reliable in the vast majority of cases, and is still the only acceptable criteria for diagnosis.

That Hirschsprung's disease might encompass a spectrum that includes hypoganglionosis, is an attractive but highly controversial theory [15].

5. Conclusion

Congenital aganglionosis presents abnormalities of defaecation from birth, and early diagnosis is possible when the clinician realises the limitations of all methods of diagnosis, but their overall potential when considered together.

Classic Hirschsprung's disease is the short segment variety, and may differ considerably in aetiology and presentation from total colonic aganglionosis.

If ultrashort segment varieties exist they are not diagnosable radiologically or histologically in the neonatal period.

Modern views emphasise the functional activity of the infiltrating abnormal nerve fibres in addition to the aganglionosis as the cause of the obstruction.

Most cases should be diagnosed in the neonatal period, and diagnostic accuracy is improved when the radiologist is alerted to the condition by clinical history and the survey radiograph. The enema technique requires limited filling and must not be hurried. Manometry also needs patience and skill, and the services of an informed pathologist are mandatory.

5.1. Acknowledgements

The authors would like to acknowledge the help and cooperation they have received from their surgical colleagues, in particular Professors J. Louw and S. Cywes. Acknowledgement to Butterworths for republishing Figure 5 from *Radiological diagnosis of digestive tract disorders in the newborn: A guide to radiologists, surgeons and paediatricians*, to the British Journal of Radiology for republishing Figures 6 and 7, and to the Journal of Pediatric Surgery for Figure 8.

References

1. BAUMGARTEN, H. G., HOLSTEIN, A. F., STELZNER, F.: Nervous elements in the human colon of Hirschsprung's disease. Virchows Arch. path. Anat. **358**, 113 (1973)
2. BERDON, W. E., BAKER, D. H.: The roentgenographic diagnosis of Hirschsprung's disease in infancy. Amer. J. Roentgenol. **93**, 432 (1965)
3. BOSTON, V. E., SCOTT, J. E. S.: Anorectal Manometry as a diagnostic method in the neonatal period. J. pediat. Surg. **11**, 9 (1976)
4. BUGHAIGHIS, A. G., EMERY, J. L.: Functional obstruction of the intestine due to neurological immaturity. Progr. pediat. Surg. **3**, 52 (1971)
5. BURNSTOCK, G.: Purinergic nerves. Pharmacol. Rev. **24**, 509 (1972)
6. CANNON, W. B.: A law of denervation. Amer. J. med. Sci. **198**, 737 (1939)
7. CHANDLER, N. W., ZWIREN, G. T.: Complete reflux of the small bowel of total colon Hirschsprung's disease. Radiology. **94**, 335 (1970)
8. CHRISTENSEN, J.: The controls of gastrointestinal movements. Some old and new views. New Engl. J. Med. **285**, 85 (1971)
9. CREMIN, B. J.: The early diagnosis of Hirschsprung's disease. Pediat. Radiol. **2**, 23 (1974)
10. CREMIN, B. J., CYWES, S., LOUW, J. H.: Radiological Diagnosis of Digestive Tract Disorders in the Newborn. A Guide to Radiologists, Surgeons and Paediatricians. London: Butterworth & Co. (1973)
11. CREMIN, B. J., GOLDING, R. L.: Congenital aganglionosis of the entire colon in neonates. Brit. J. Radiol. **49**, 27 (1976)
12. DAVIS, W. S., ALLAN, R. P., FAVARA, B. E.: Neonatal small left colon synchome. Amer. J. Roentgenol. **120**, 322 (1974)
13. DEFFRENNE, P., DAUDET, M., CHAPPUIS, J. P.: Radiological diagnosis of total aganglionosis of the colon. Ann. Radiol. **14**, 357 (1971)
14. EHRENPREIS, T.: Hirschsprung's disease. Year Book Medical Publishers Inc. Chicago. **62**, 81 (1970)
15. EMERY, J. L.: (Personal Communication). (1976)
16. FRECH, R. S.: Aganglionosis involving the entire colon and a variable length of small bowel. Radiology. **90**, 249 (1968)
17. GOWERS, W. R.: The autonomic action of the sphincter ani. Proc. Roy. Soc. Lond. **26**, 77 (1878)
18. HIRSCHSPRUNG, H.: Stuhlträgheit Neugeborener in Folge von Dilatation und Hypertrophie des Colons. Jb. Kinderheilk. N.F. **XXVII**, 1 (1888)
19. HOPE, J. W., BORNS, P. F., BERG, P. K.: Roentgenologic manifestations of Hirschsprung's disease in infancy. Amer. J. Roentgenol. **95**, 217 (1965)
20. HOWARD, R. R., NIXON, H. H.: The internal anal sphincter—observation on development and mechanism of inhibitory responses in premature infants and children with H.D. Arch. Dis. Childh. **43**, 569 (1968)
21. LAWSON, J. O. N., NIXON, H. H.: Anal canal pressure in the diagnosis of H.D. J. pediat. Surg. **2**, 544 (1967)
22. MEIER-RUGE, W., LUTTERBECK, P. M., HERTZOG, B., MORGER, R., MOSER, R., SCHARLI, A.: Acetylcholinesterase activity in suction biopsies of the rectum in the diagnosis of Hirschsprung's disease. J. pediat. Surg. **7**, 11 (1972)
23. NOBLETT, H. R.: A rectal suction biopsy tube for use in the diagnosis of Hirschsprung's disease. J. pediat. Surg. **4**, 486 (1969)

24. OKAMOTO, E., UEDA, T.: Embryogenesis of intramural ganglia of the gut and its relation to Hirschsprung's disease. J. pediat. Surg. **2**, 437 (1967)

25. RUYSCH, F.: Observationum Anatomica Chirurgi-
carum Centuria (1691). Quoted by LEENDERS, E.,
and SIEBER, W. K. J. pediat. Surg. **5**, 1 (1970)

26. SCHNAUFER, L.,   TALBERT, J. L.,   HALLER, J. A.,
REID, N. C. S. W., TOBON, F., SCHUSTER, M. M.: Differential sphinteric studies in the diagnosis of anorectal disorders of childhood. J. pediat. Surg. **2**, 538
(1967)

27. SMITH, B.: Neuropathology of the Alimentary
Tract. London: Edward Arnold Publishers. 1972,
p. 14

28. TIFFIN, M. E., CHANDLER, L. R., FABER, H. K.: Localised absence of the ganglion cells of the myen-
teric plexus in congenital megacolon. Amer. J. Dis.
Childh. **59**, 1071 (1940)

29. WOOD, J. D.: Neurophysiology of Auerbach's
Plexus and control of intestinal motility. Physiol.
Rev. **55**, 307 (1975)

Renal Cysts and Cystlike Conditions in Infancy and Childhood

C. Fauré

1. Introduction

If we accepted as a cyst only a cavity filled with clear fluid, interiorly lined by epithelium, located in the renal parenchyma, and which does not communicate with the excretory ducts and cavities, we should accept only a few entities. Unfortunately, the term cyst has been applied to several diseases in which cavities or holes are found in the renal substance, sometimes communicating with the renal cavities. A confusion in terminology renders the problem even more complex. It is not

Table 1. Classification of renal cysts

I. Renal dysplasia
A. Multicystic kidney
B. Focal and segmental cystic dysplasia
C. Multiple cysts associatied with lower urinary tract obstruction
D. Familial cystic dysplasia

II. Hereditary cystic diseases
A. Medullary cystic disease (nephronophthisis)
B. Zellweger's cerebrohepatorenal syndrome
C. Jeune's asphyxiating dystrophy
D. Meckel's syndrome
E. Tuberous sclerosis complex and Lindau's disease
F. Hepatorenal polycystic disease:
    infantile form
    juvenile form
    adult form

III. Miscellaneous
Trisomy cysts
Simple cysts, solitary and multiple
Multilocular cysts
Medullary sponge kidney
Pyelogenic cyst and calyceal diverticulum
Parapelvic cyst
Perinephric cyst
Echinococcal cyst

Modified from R. HABIB and from J. BERNSTEIN.

uncommon to find a report describing a condition in terms which, in another classification, refer to an entirely different entity. For instance, the term "sponge kidney" in an infant is sometimes used to describe a case of infantile polycystic disease, whereas it should in fact refer only to the medullary sponge kidney disease described by CACCHI and RICCI [3], and LINDVALL [16].

There is unfortunately no reliable criterion to be drawn from the domain of etiopathogeny, or from that of a specific embryologic defect, or from histologic appearance, or from the roentgenologic features, which establishes a logical classification. Personally, we think that in dealing with such a topic we must describe several well-established entities, giving the proper term and the synonyms used for each of them. There are several ways to present these diseases. We use a classification established by HABIB [12] working with a team of pediatric nephrologists, urologists and radiologists and modified from BERNSTEIN [1] (Table 1). First, we shall study the dysplastic cystic diseases.

2. The Multicystic Kidney

(Multicystic renal dysplasia, unilateral total renal dysplasia)
This term refers to a severely dysplastic cystic kidney. The lesion, as a rule unilateral, is macroscopically characterized by a bunch of smooth, thin-walled cysts (Fig. 1) of varying sizes and filled with clear fluid. No renal parenchyma is visible from the outer surface; the cysts are connected by apparently fibrous tissue. The ureter is almost always absent or atretic for a part of its course, and the kidney pelvis is also atretic, as stressed by

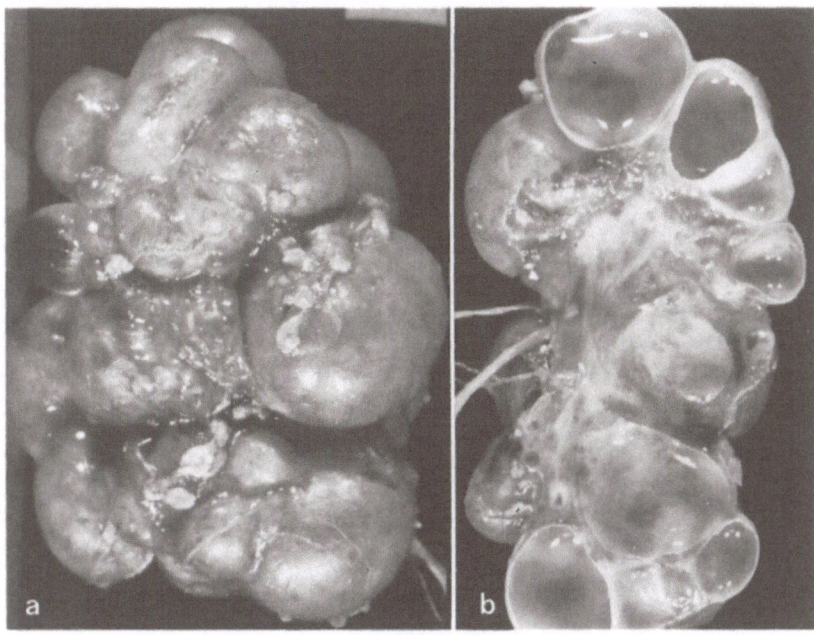

Fig. 1 a and b. External a) and cut b) appearances of a multicystic kidney

GRISCOM et al. [10]. The renal artery is absent or diminutive and sometimes does not follow its usual course.

Histologically, the tissue around the cysts is composed of bands of a fibrous or embryonic stroma containing immature glomeruli, primitive tubules, smooth muscle cells, and occasional islands of cartilage. The cysts are lined by a flattened epithelium. Other congenital malformations have been seen in association with this anomaly. The liver as a rule is normal. The condition is rarely bilateral, but if it is it is lethal. This congenital anomaly is not hereditary or familial though cases have been noted in twins.

Usually discovered during the first weeks or months of life, the multicystic kidney commonly presents itself as a mass in the flank. According to GRISCOM et al. [10], it is the most frequent etiology of the lumboabdominal masses discovered during the first 2 days of life. Abdominal pain and failure to thrive are sometimes noted. Unless there is obstruction or hydronephrosis of the other kidney, urinanalysis is normal. Plain roentgenograms of the abdomen show a large area of aqueous density in the flank, displacing the gas-containing bowel. In rare cases, in older children, ringlike calcifications are identified within the mass.

During excretory pyelography the unaffected kidney appears normal or shows compensatory hypertrophy, while there is failure to visualize any renal cavities on the involved side, even hours after injection. Nevertheless with the high dose of contrast now used for intravenous pyelography (IVP) in infants and children, it is fairly common to see within the mass, after a few minutes, faint thin curvilinear shadows around circular or oval lucencies. This septation sign (Fig. 2) is of great diagnostic value, but its pathogenesis is not clear. Is it, as stated by many authors, a manifestation of the total body opacification in the walls of the cysts? Is it, as suggested by others, a faint excretion of the contrast medium by a few remaining functional glomeruli and tubules? This is the opinion of DOBERTI and ESCUDERO [4]. FELSON [7] stresses the fact that this sign may be found even when low doses are used, and that it may persist even after half an hour. Also of interest is the observation related by YOUNG et al. [18] who found a puddling of contrast medium within the cyst lumens 24 or 48 h after IVP. These facts seem

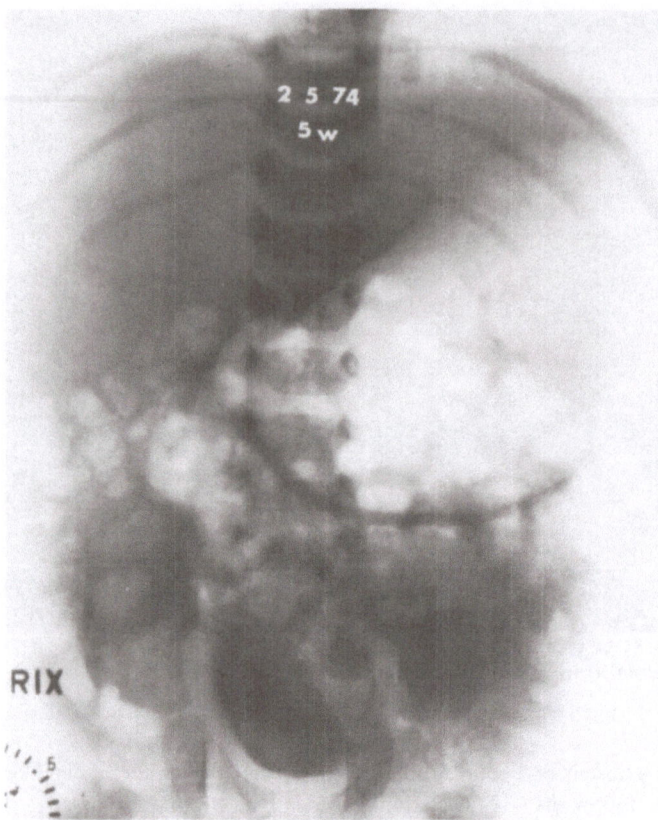

Fig. 2. Right multicystic kidney in a 5-week-old infant (same case as Fig. 1). On the five minute IVP film there is no secretion on the right side, but septal walls are seen encircling round or oval lucencies superimposed on the liver opacity

to corroborate the view expressed by FELSON and CUSSEN [8] that multicystic disease represents hydronephrosis secondary to atresia of the ureter or of the pelvis or of both, during the metanephric stage of intrauterine development.

GRISCOM et al. [10] do not accept this theory and consider that forms in which the cysts communicate with each other and with a large pelvis are malformed embryonic hydronephroses, even if there are associated criteria of dysplasia.

Other radiologic findings are of less interest: The atretic ureter may be shown by retrograde pyelography. However, this investigation has sometimes resulted in a perforation of this cul-de-sac and should be avoided. An absent or minute renal artery may be shown by abdominal aortography but this examination is usually not necessary. In difficult cases, echotomography may be helpful. The radiologic signs permit us to differentiate the multicystic kidney from Wilm's tumor, renal ha-martoma (Bolande's tumor), unilateral renal vein thrombosis and hydronephrosis. In the latter, crescentic opaque lines may be seen, but after several hours a faint opacification of the dilated cavities is obtained. The diagnosis is more difficult in very severe hydronephrosis but this will be only a matter of nosology if we accept Felson's theory for the multicystic kidney.

Nevertheless in both cases surgical removal is the only treatment after it is established that the other kidney is functioning. The prognosis is good, though the other kidney is sometimes hydronephrotic and this may require treatment.

Other Varieties of Cystic Dysplasia. Cystic dysplasia may be associated with low *urinary tract obstruction*. This obstruction, commonly posterior urethral valves in boys, leads to a severe bilateral hydronephrosis and hydroureter, which is seen on IVP films but usually obscures the changes suggestive of cystic dysplasia. This condition is discovered during surgery or more often at post-mortem examination. Such dysplastic cysts are often seen in the parenchyma of the upper component of a duplicated kidney affected by ureterocele. *Focal segmental dysplasia* rarely occurs, and when discovered can suggest other entities such as cystadenoma. *Hypoplasia with diffuse cystic dysplasia* is a rare entity which appears as renal insufficiency and acidosis. According to HABIB [12], this variety probably includes cases of familial hepatorenal cystic dysplasia (see below).

3. Familial Cystic Renal Conditions

Among familial cystic renal conditions, some deserve only brief comment:
Medullary cystic disease, also called *nephronophthisis* is transmitted as an autosomal trait, sometimes recessive, sometimes dominant. It is predominantly encountered in children and young adults. It is characterized by anemia, saltwasting, polyuria and progressive renal insufficiency. Tapeto-retinal degeneration is sometimes associated. The intravenous urogram shows relatively small kidneys, with poorly concentrated contrast. High dosage nephrotomography may disclose well-defined corticomedullary lucencies, suggesting the presence of cysts. Medullary tubular ectasia is a quite common finding but usually appears only by retrograde pyelography which may sometimes also inject the cysts. Renal arteriography is the most valuable investigation, showing the renal atrophy to be mainly cortical, and the presence of cysts. However, renal biopsy is often necessary to establish the diagnosis.
In the *hepatocerebrorenal syndrome* renal cysts, usually glomerular, are a common histologic finding, but without radiologic expression. In the same way, the *microcystic renal disease*, which characterizes some familial nephrotic syndromes, usually only concerns the pathologist.
Jeune's asphyxiating thoracic dysplasia includes renal abnormalities, the most severe of which is a type of dysplasia; in the least severe form the renal cortex is scattered with microcysts of trivial inter-

est to the radiologist. *Meckel's syndrome* of cerebral maldevelopment may include cysts in greatly enlarged kidneys. In *Laurence-Moon-Biedl's disease* tubular precalyceal ectasia and even calyceal diverticula may be observed in normal- or small-sized kidneys.
The renal lesions of *tuberous sclerosis* are as a rule multiple hamartomas. However, multiple true cysts may be observed, sometimes leading to renal insufficiency, as shown in Figure 3 in the case of a 6-month-old infant. Roentgenologically, they give the same appearance as adult polycystic disease, with lucencies in the cortical nephrogram shown on nephrotomography or arteriography.

Among the familial hereditary cystic diseases, the most important are the hepatorenal *polycystic diseases* which appear in four varieties.
Adult polycystic kidney disease is inherited as an autosomal dominant trait with a high penetrance, without sex predilection. It is characterized pathologically by an important enlargement of the kidney, bilateral but often asymmetrical. Variable-sized cysts, located in both medulla and cortex, bulge under the capsule separated by bands of normal renal tissue. Hepatic cysts occur in approximately a third of the patients, but usually without periportal fibrosis. Cysts may be found in pancreas, lungs, spleen, ovaries, testes, etc., and in 11% of cases a berry aneurysm of intracranial arteries is present, at least in adults.
Although it is relatively common, since the incidence ranges from 1 per 350 to 1 per 620 in necropsy material, it is extremely rare during an IVP in a child to encounter a well-developed form with enlarged kidneys and grossly distorted and stretched calyces and pelvis (Fig. 4a). Nephrography reveals the cysts as lucencies. In such cases, one must always verify that one is not dealing with a case of tuberous sclerosis.

As a rule the disease remains clinically and even radiologically silent until 40 or 50 years of age. Even in affected families urographic examinations fail to detect the disease until adulthood. For early detection, nephrotomography or angiography are the best investigations. They may show a Swisscheese appearance of the cortical nephrogram but this sign is not always present at an early phase in patients who will present with poly-

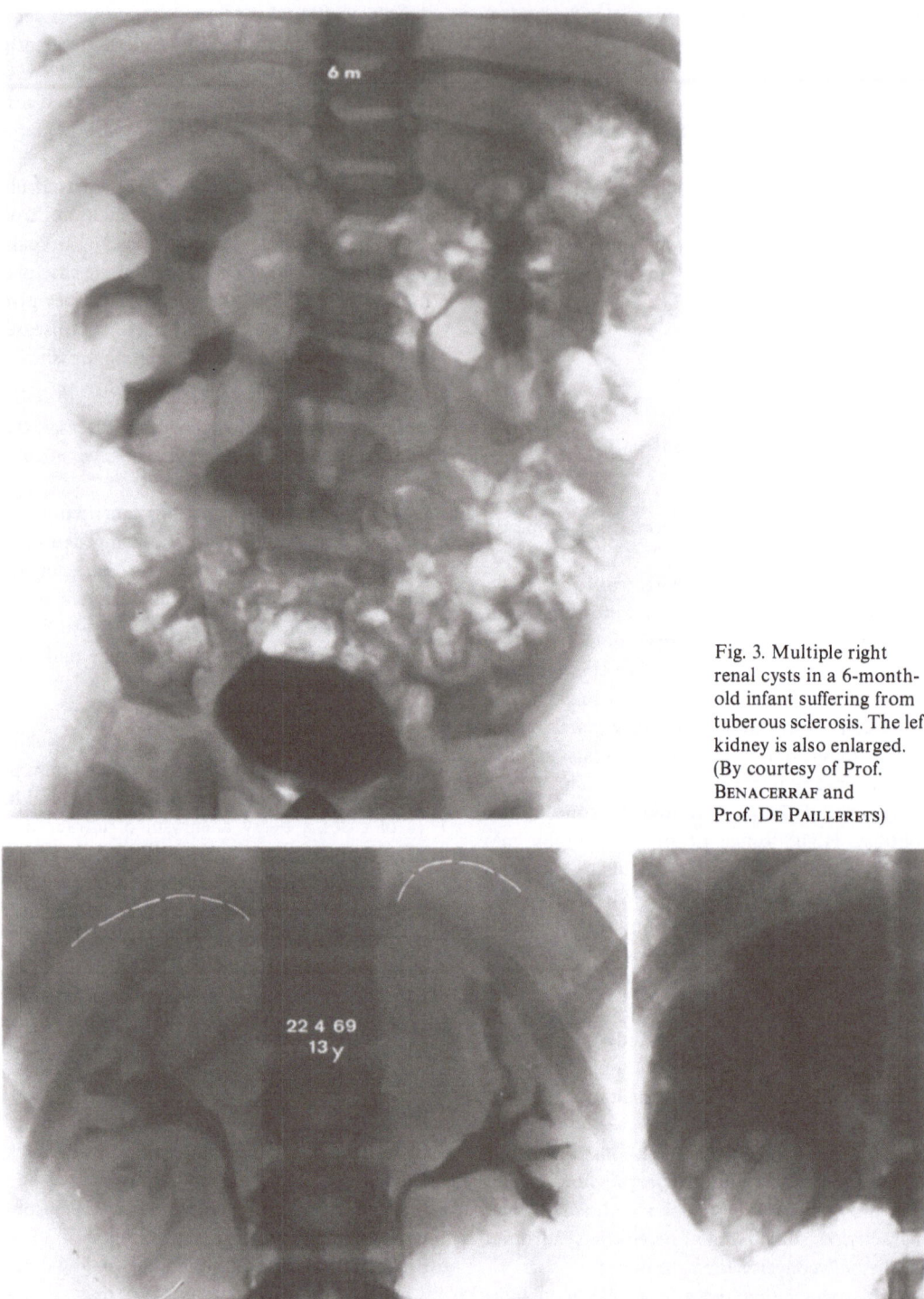

Fig. 3. Multiple right
renal cysts in a 6-month-
old infant suffering from
tuberous sclerosis. The left
kidney is also enlarged.
(By courtesy of Prof.
BENACERRAF and
Prof. DE PAILLERETS)

Fig. 4a and b. Dominant polycystic disease of the kidneys in a 13-year-old girl. a) Urographic appearance.

b) Nephrographic phase of aortography showing multiple round lucencies in the right kidney

cystic kidneys. Nevertheless well-advanced forms have been reported in infants. Prognosis is obviously very poor when the disease is symptomatic in a child.

Infantile polycystic disease of the kidneys (IPCD) [1] is uncommon, occuring in 1 per 6000 to 1 per 14000 births, more commonly in females. It is inherited as an autosomal recessive trait. Pathological findings are characteristic. Macroscopically both kidneys are bilaterally tremendously enlarged. The kidneys keep their general shape, with lobulation, and tiny cysts stud the outer surface. The cut surface has a spongy or a honeycomb appearance involving both cortex and medulla (Fig. 5). Microscopically the cysts are seen to represent dilated tubules and nephrons throughout the cortex, the medulla and papilla. The liver in almost all cases is enlarged with multiple tiny hepatic cysts, periportal fibrosis and dilated bile ductules. Associated anomalies have been described but, according to LIEBERMAN and coworkers [15] they are probably fortuitous associations or acquired lesions. The urinary tract is otherwise normal.

Clinical presentation is variable:
1. It may be discovered on autopsy in a stillborn.
2. The huge kidneys may obstruct delivery.
3. In the majority of cases, the disease manifests itself in the first days or weeks of life by flank masses in an infant with renal insufficiency; the liver is generally enlarged.
4. Some patients have a Potter's facies.
5. Several cases are discovered because of neonatal respiratory distress due to pneumothorax or pneumomediastinum.
6. Left ventricular hypertrophy with cardiac failure may occur.
7. In affected families the prenatal diagnosis may be roentgenologically suspected on a general deflexion of the fetal spine.

The roentgenographic findings are characteristic: On the plain film, the enlarged kidneys appear as large areas of aqueous density displacing the bowel gas.

---

[1] (Infantile polycystic disease of the kidneys and liver is the proper term; the others, such as hamartomatous cystic kidneys, infantile sponge kidney, lead to confusion, and must be dropped).

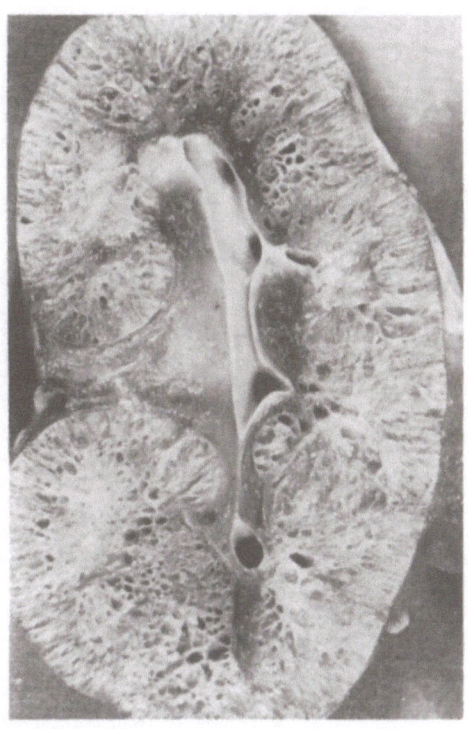

Fig. 5. Infantile polycystic disease. Cut appearance of the kidney

In the IVP (Fig. 6) the nephrogram is delayed but is usually prolonged. Progressively, superimposed on the nephrogram, appear faint streaks of contrast giving these huge kidneys a mottled or streaky pattern. This pattern is reinforced in a brush-border appearance near the calyces in the papillae. The calyces and the pelvis, poorly opacified due to the lack of concentration appear stretched and distorted. This picture is often more clearly visible in tomograms. The kidneys retain the contrast medium for hours or even days. Renal arteriography is of no use; and, while a retrograde pyelogram may better visualize the pelvi-calyceal systems and the reflux in ectatic tubules, it is a dangerous procedure that has led to serious complications in some cases. The diagnosis is easy: bilateral Wilms' tumor, hydronephrosis or multicystic kidney can be ruled out on the basis of the urographic appearance. The prognosis is very poor: the infant usually dies during the first weeks or months. Survival past infancy is rare, but has been reported.

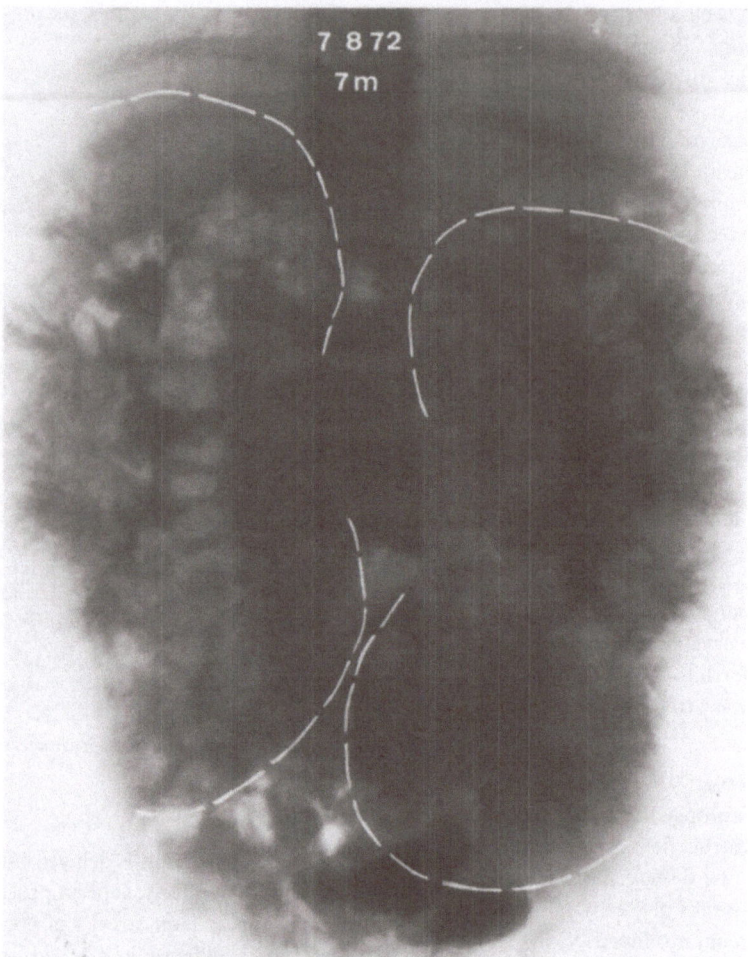

Fig. 6. Urographic (3 h film) pattern of infantile polycystic disease in a 7-month-old boy

Childhood or juvenile polycystic disease of the kidneys is inherited as an autosomal recessive trait without sex predilection. In this variety, the renal component is moderate and the liver involvement more conspicuous. Pathologically, the kidneys are moderately enlarged, but keep their shape (Fig. 7); the cysts are fewer in number, and specifically located in the medulla, where one can see some tiny cysts and medullary tubular ectasia: on the postmortem specimen of Figure 8, in which pelvis and calyces have been injected as well as arteries, the tubular ectasia is visible. Hepatomegaly is quite constant; there is an important periportal fibrosis and an abnormal development of the interlobular bile ducts leads to saccular dilatation of the biliary tree. Associated malformations are frequent, such as harelips, hamartoma of the third ventricle, inferior vena cava stenosis, choledocal cyst, etc.

Clinically the onset of the disease takes place in late childhood at about 9 years of age on the average. The clinical manifestations are usually portal hypertension with digestive tract bleeding, hepatosplenomegaly, sometimes angiocholitis. Kidney involvement as a rule remains clinically silent. Roentgenologically the plain abdominal films show enlarged liver and spleen, and normal or slightly enlarged kidneys.

Excretory urography usually shows blunt papillae, and medullary tubular ectasia is a fairly com-

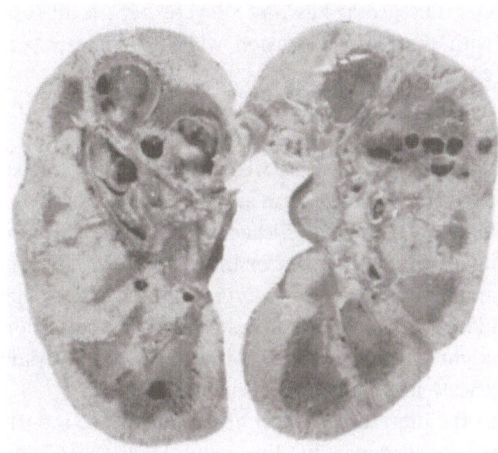

Fig. 7. Cut appearance of a kidney affected by juvenile polycystic disease

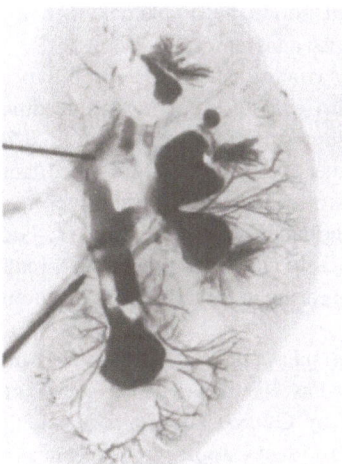

Fig. 8. Autopsy specimen of juvenile polycystic kidney after injection of arteries and renal cavities. The tubular ectasia is quite visible

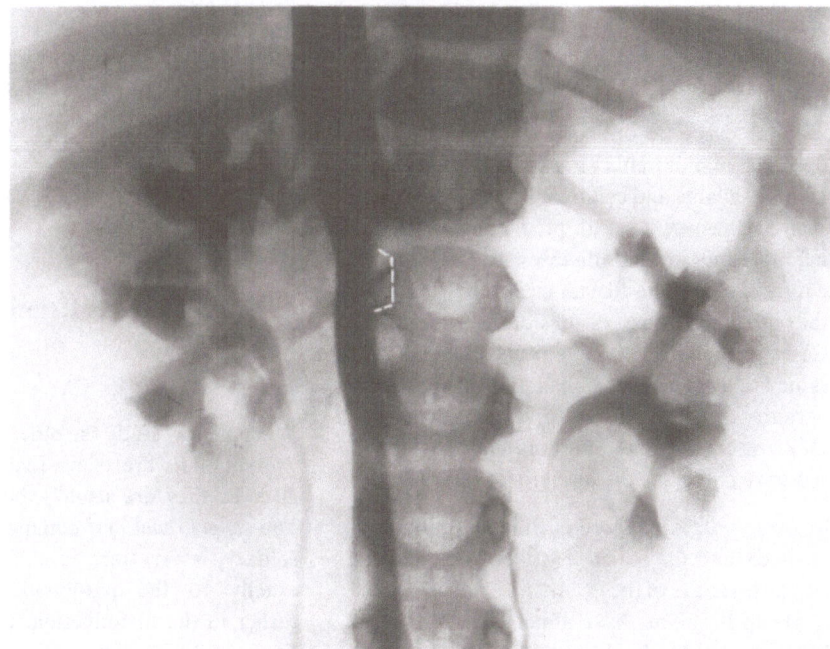

Fig. 9. Juvenile polycystic disease of the kidneys. Urographic appearance during a caval phlebography for assessment of a mesenterico-caval anastomosis

mon finding, as in the child of Figure 9, whose kidneys are opacified during a control examination after a mesenterico-caval anastomosis. The child recovered, and the urographic appearance 11 years later is shown. The pelvicalyceal systems are otherwise normal or slightly stretched but never as distorted as in the adult polycystic disease. Parenchymal cysts may be seen on nephrotomograms. Renal arteriography is in our opinion not necessary.

Esophageal varices are usually present, detected by barium investigation. Splenoportography, when performed, shows hepatic block with numerous portocaval anastomoses.

The prognosis is conditioned by the portal hypertension and the risk of cataclysmic bleeding. Death may also result from angiocholitis. The kidney involvement is usually well tolerated, and even in patients operated on for portal hypertension it may never manifest itself, or only very late. However, a few cases have been related with renal insufficiency appearing in the adolescent or young adult.

Familial cystic dysplasia of liver and kidneys is the fourth entity. It has been described by IVEMARK et al. [14] and by GWINN and LANDING [11]. During IVP the kidneys appear to be enlarged with tubular ectasia. The liver is enlarged. The reality of this entity is disputed. It probably encompasses familial disorders with kidney cysts such as Jeune's, or Zellweger's, or Laurence-Moon-Biedl's diseases.

Let us now turn to the first three varieties of *hepatorenal polycystic diseases*. Everybody does accept the existence of a dominant disease, rarely observed in children, and a recessive form which involves infants and children. But if some authors, such as LIEBERMAN et al. [15], consider that the infantile and juvenile diseases are two different entities, others like ROYER et al. [17] think that they are different expressions of the same disease. Cases of each variety have been observed in the same family. The best explanation of the various patterns of the disease is given by BLYTH and OCKENDEN [2]. These authors have divided the recessive polycystic disease into four groups.

In group I, 90% or more of the renal tubules are involved, and the patient is stillborn or dies during the first days of life.

In group II, infants have about 60% of their tubules affected by the disease; they live somewhat longer, until the first or second year of life.

In group III, infants have about 25% of their tubules affected by the disease; they live longer than the other groups, sometimes without or only with late renal troubles; they may show signs of hepatic fibrosis and eventually die from complications of this liver disease.

In group IV, the patients have only about 10% of their kidneys involved by the cystic process. However this group has more severe hepatic fibrosis with portal hypertension which dominates and conditions the prognosis.

So groups I and II fit in with the infantile form, groups III and IV with the juvenile form.

We may also discuss what the relations are between the infantile form and the medullary sponge kidney. DUTRUGE [5] has related the case of an infant who died from infantile polycystic disease and whose father has a typical medullary sponge kidney, and she has suggested that this condition might be the expression of the recessive polycystic disease in a heterozygote carrier.

In the literature, several observations are reported, for instance by EBEL and OLBING [6], by HOEFFEL and coworkers [13a,b], by GAISFORD and BLOOR [9], which do not fit into any classification. Consequently, we must study more deeply these polycystic renal diseases and try to find out if there are links between the adult dominant and child or infant recessive forms. But to go further in that direction, we can take into account only well-documented cases, with data about family history, genetic transmission, gross and microscopic pathology, clinical and radiological symptoms.

4. Miscellaneous Renal Cystic Conditions

We shall now study the other cystic diseases:
Trisomy cysts are of no real interest to radiologists, as they are usually post-mortem findings. The *simple renal cyst* commonly, but not always, solitary, is very rare in children. It corresponds exactly to the pathological definition given earlier in the introduction. Clinically discovered as an abdominal mass, it appears during intravenous urography as an expansive process within the kidney and always raises the diagnosis of nephroblastoma; commonly, with a high dose of contrast, a round lucency appears in the nephrogram, sometimes limited by a thin opaque rim. When some doubt remains it is necessary to confirm the diagnosis by renal arteriography. Echotomography is also of great importance for differentiating a cyst from a Wilms' tumor.

Renal multilocular cyst or cystadenoma is a rare benign condition but perhaps more frequent than the solitary cyst. Pathologically (Fig. 10), it is a well-limited lesion in which numerous juxtaposed cysts are separated by connective walls containing smooth muscle cells and sometimes dysplastic glomerulo-tubular structures. The noninvolved renal parenchyma is normal.

Radiologically (Fig. 11) the cystadenoma appears as a renal expansive process. Renal arteriography shows (Fig. 11) a peculiar appearance with the walls of the cysts appearing within the lucency of the tumoral mass. In several reported cases abnormal vessels have been seen in the tumor and differentiation from nephroblastoma was arrived at only after surgery, by gross and histological examination.

The exact nature of this entity has been disputed. There are certainly cases which border on cystic dysplasia and others on cystic nephroblastoma.

Medullary sponge kidney or CACCHI and RICCI's disease, though of congenital origin, is extremely rare in children. Pathologically it is characterized by the presence of tiny cavities, in the medullary pyramids and papillae giving them, when cut, a spongy appearance. The number of cysts and their extension into the pyramids are quite variable. They often contain calculi. These cysts are represented by enlarged papillary ducts or in other words by precalyceal tubular ectasia. The lesion is isolated. The kidneys are of normal size. There is no associated hepatic involvement; cases reported with bile duct enlargement belong, in our opinion, to juvenile polycystic disease.

The diagnosis is made by roentgen examination; small round calculi are sometimes present, scattered in several papillae. Intravenous urography shows calyces with blunt and enlarged papillae, and, inside the papillae, several small round or elongated cavities, clustered in a "branch of flowers" which represent tubular ectasia.

So rare is the disease in children that one must always verify that one is not dealing with a precalyceal physiologic blur or with a condition simulating tubular ectasia such as renal tuberculosis, papillary necrosis which can appear in diabetes mellitus or sickle-cell anemia, or as kidney lesions of Laurence-Moon-Biedl disease. If tubular ecta-

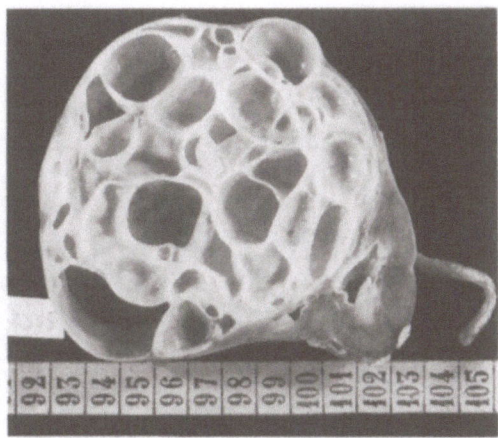

Fig. 10. Cut appearance of cystadenoma of the kidney

sia is confirmed one must remember that this finding is not an entity per se, but is a syndrome found in other conditions such as nephronophthisis or juvenile polycystic disease. Such findings in a child must lead to an esophageal barium examination, looking for varices, and even to percutaneous liver biopsy in search of hepatic fibrosis.

Pyelogenic cyst and calyceal diverticulum are quite similar lesions rarely encountered in children. At intravenous urography, they appear as a small round cavity in the renal parenchyma near a calyx communicating with it by a narrow isthmus. *Parapelvic cyst*, a rare condition in the adult, is not known in children. *Pararenal pseudocyst* is a fibrous encapsulation of extravasated urine, commonly under the capsula; of traumatic origin, it is sometimes observed in childhood but is not really a cyst. In the same way, we cannot consider as true cysts cavitation which takes place after pyogenic suppuration, tuberculosis caseation or tumoral necrosis.

Renal cyst is a rare localization of echinococcus disease; when not ruptured, it presents itself like any simple cyst. When the external and not the internal layer of the cyst is ruptured, contrast may infiltrate from the calyx around the cyst. When all layers are ruptured, the cyst cavity is opacified through the calyx.

Such are the different varieties of cystic or cystlike conditions involving the kidneys in infancy and childhood. I hope this will provide the basis of a better approach to these diseases.

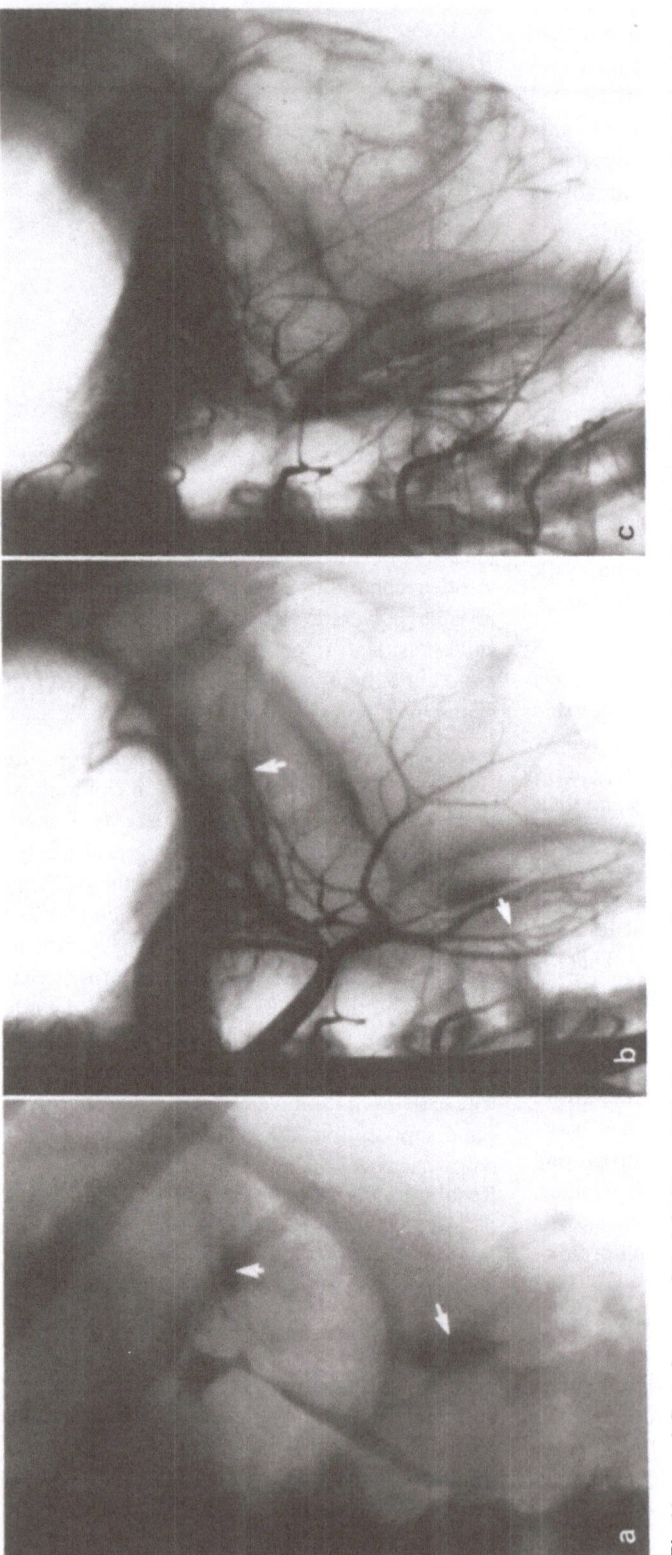

Fig. 11a—c. a) Cystadenoma of the left kidney. IVP showing an expanding lesion of the lower pole. Arteriography showing displacement of vessels around the lesion b) and walls of the cysts faintly opacified within the lucency of the tumoral mass c)

References

1. BERNSTEIN, J.: The classification of renal cysts. Nephron 11, 91—100 (1973)
2. BLYTH, H., OCKENDEN, B.: Polycystic disease of kidneys and liver presenting in childhood. J. Med. Genet. 8, 257—284 (1971)
3. CACCHI, R., RICCI, V.: Sopra une rara e forse non ancore descritta affezione cistica delle piramidi renali (rene a spugna). 21 Congresso della Soc. Ital. di Urologia, Bologna, 1948
4. DOBERTI, B. A., ESCUDERO, G.: Riñon multiquistico y hemorragia suprarenales del recien nacido. Rev. Interamer. Rad. 2, 24—35 (1967)
5. DUTRUGE, J.: Contribution à l'étude de la polykystose hépato-rénale chez le nourrisson et l'enfant. (A propos de huit observations personnelles associant fibro-adénomatose biliaire et reins polykystiques). Thesis, Lyon, 1969
6. EBEL, K., OLBING, H.: Zur Röntendiagnostik der polyzistischen Nierendegeneration im Kindesalter. Fortschr. Röntgenstr. 110, 28—38 (1969)
7. FELSON, B.: Letter from the editor. Seminars Roentgenol. 10, 93—94 (1975)
8. FELSON, B., CUSSEN, L. J.: The hydronephrotic type of unilateral congenital multicystic disease of the kidney. Seminars Roentgenol. 10, 113—123 (1975)
9. GAISFORD, W., BLOOR, K.: Congenital polycystic disease of the kidneys and liver. Portal hypertension. Porto-caval anastomosis. Proc. roy. Soc. Med. 61, 304—305 (1968)
10. GRISCOM, N. T., VAWTER, G. F., FELLERS, F. X.: Pelvoinfundibular atresia: The usual form of multicystic kidney: 44 unilateral and two bilateral cases. Seminars Roentgenol. 10, 125—131 (1975)
11. GWINN, J. L., LANDING, B. H.: Cystic diseases of the kidneys in infants and children. Radiologic Clinics of North America VI-2, 191—204 (1968)
12. HABIB, R.: Renal dysplasia, hypoplasia and cysts. Pediat. Nephrol. 1, 209—229 (1974)
13a. HOEFFEL, J. C.: Classification of renal cysts in children. Aust. Radiol. 14, 302—307 (1970)
13b. HOEFFEL, J. C., BOURGEOIS, J. M., JACOTTIN, G.: Classification des kystes du rein chez l'enfant. Ouest Médical 23, 135—142 (1970)
14. IVEMARK, B. I., OLDFELT, V., ZETTERSTROM, R.: Familial dysplasia of kidneys, liver and pancreas; a probably genetically determined syndrome. Acta Paediat. 48, 1—11 (1959)
15. LIEBERMAN, E., SALINAS-MADRIGAL, L., GWINN, J. L., BRENNAN, L. P., FINE, R. N., LANDING, B. H.: Infantile polycystic disease of the kidneys and liver: Clinical, pathological and radiological correlations and comparison with congenital hepatic fibrosis. Medicine 50, 277—318 (1971)
16. LINDVALL, N.: Roentgenologic diagnosis of medullary sponge kidney. Acta Radiol. 51 193—206 (1959)
17. ROYER, P., FREZAL, J., BOIS, E., FEINGOLD, J.: Les néphropathies héréditaires. Arch. franç. Pédiat. 27, 293—317 (1970)
18. YOUNG, L. W., WOOD, B. P., SPOHR, C. H., PANNER, B.: Delayed excretory urographic opacification, a puddling effect, in multicystic renal dysplasia. Ann. Radiol. 17, 391—396 (1974)

Aspects of Acute Kidney Injury in Young Infants

A. R. Chrispin

1. Introduction

This report is concerned primarily with the impact of the shock state on the kidney. When cardiac output falls, renal blood flow and renal parenchymal nutrition are affected. The clinical circumstances which may lead to a shock state in young infants are noted. Clinical features and radiological findings in such kidney lesions as tubular necrosis, medullary necrosis, and renal venous thrombosis are described. Although the kidney of the young infant is especially vulnerable there has been some evidence of concomitant damage to other organs, namely, the adrenals and brain.

2. The Kidney and the Shock State

2.1. Pathological Types of Kidney Injury

There are certain types of acute kidney damage which are caused neither by direct trauma nor by acute infection. These forms of kidney damage include cortical necrosis, medullary necrosis, tubular necrosis and renal venous thrombosis.

This survey is concerned with infants under the age of 4 months who have medullary and tubular necrosis: these two conditions commonly occur at the same time in the same infant. The survey is also concerned with renal venous thrombosis in young infants. In all these infants there has been reason to believe that a shock state has precipitated kidney injury.

2.2. Clinical Causes of the Shock State

Infants with these types of kidney damage have suffered primarily from what are apparently disparate clinical conditions. The antecedent illnesses are listed in Table 1.

Gastroenteritis has been by far the commonest of all these illnesses, and indeed it was present in the three infants whose clinical and radiological features formed the basis of an early report [4]. Since then further cases, having different primary conditions, have been encountered [5] and no doubt the list will continue to have further additions as time passes.

Table 1

Gastroenteritis
Neonatal hepatitis
Ventricular septal defect and anaemia
Perinatal asphyxia
Pneumonia
Maternal diabetes
Pyloric stenosis
Salicylate poisoning and hypoglycaemia

The Effect of the Shock State. Some infants have clearly been in a state of clinical shock as a consequence of the primary illness. Such a state is associated with a reduction in cardiac output. Of all the organs supplied by the systemic circulation, the kidney is perhaps especially vulnerable to a reduction in cardiac output and systemic blood flow, because it ordinarily receives such a large fraction of the cardiac output. In these young infants it may be surmised that, as cardiac output fell, renal blood flow fell very sharply. Stasis in blood circulation in the kidney will affect the nutrition and ultimately the viability of parenchymal cells. In this way renal parenchymal cell necrosis can become manifest as tubular necrosis and medullary necrosis.

In shock, the coagulability of blood increases [1]. When the blood flow is exceptionally slow there is a possibility of intravascular coagulation occurring. The long vasa recta of the medulla seem to be one site where coagulation is especially likely, and this can lead to medullary necrosis. Coagulation in small renal veins leads to tissue damage and the clinical and pathologic features of renal venous thrombosis. Later recanalisation could make recovery of renal parenchyma a possibility. However, not all these infants have been in what appears clinically as a serious state of shock. Such clinical appearances are very probably deceptive, and there is no lack of evidence to suggest this is so. Cardiac by-pass surgery quite commonly precipitates a state of reversible clinical shock in which the parameters are under surveillance: a sharply reduced cardiac output when associated with vasoconstriction need not necessarily be associated either with a fall in systemic arterial blood pressure or with an altered heart rate. Young infants are especially susceptible to shock because the extra vascular fluid compartment is relatively smaller than in later life.

3. Clinical Features and Radiological Findings in Tubular Necrosis and Medullary Necrosis

3.1. Acute Illness

Clinical Features. At the time of acute kidney damage there was usually a detectable oliguric phase lasting 2 or 3 days. Often the oliguria could reasonably be expected to have been present as part of the precipitating illness when this was, for example, gastroenteritis.

Then began the second polyuric phase. The excessive water loss was also accompanied by excessive loss of sodium and other cations: some elevation of blood urea was found. In this second phase the

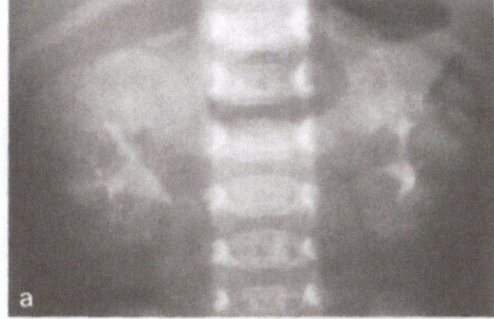
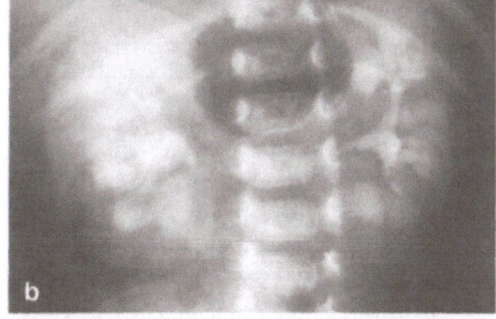

Fig. 1a—c. a) IVU 3 weeks after a Ramstedt procedure for hypertrophic pyloric stenosis. Radiograph at 5 min shows the immediate increase in overall density which is a feature of tubular necrosis. Slight increase in density of medulla is also shown

b) Same IVU as in (a). This shows marked increase in overall density of kidneys with exceptionally dense opacification of medulla (indicative of medullary necrosis) and also of cortex adjacent to cortico-medullary junction

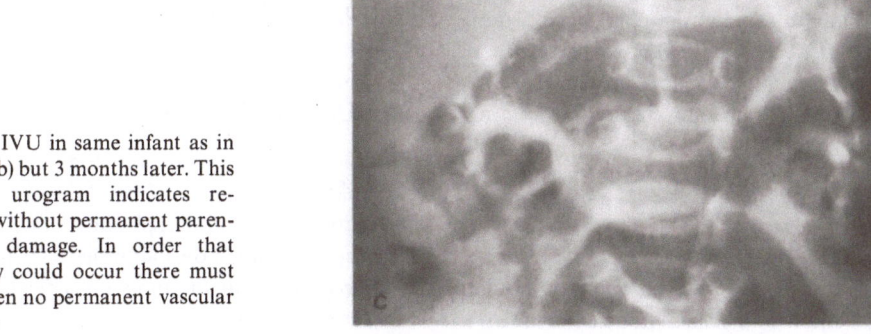

Fig. 1c. IVU in same infant as in (a) and (b) but 3 months later. This normal urogram indicates recovery without permanent parenchymal damage. In order that recovery could occur there must have been no permanent vascular damage

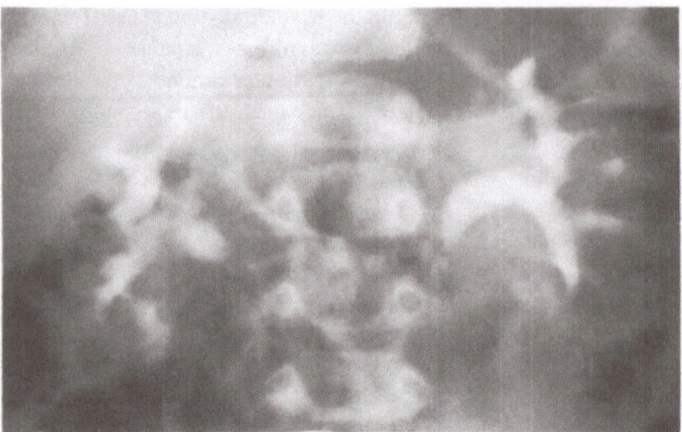

Fig. 2. IVU in an infant who 3 months previously had an IVU with similar features to those shown in Figures 1a and b. Tubular necrosis was proved on a cortical biopsy. Permanent and irrecoverable medullary necrosis is shown by widespread caliectasis, indicating complete loss of renal papillae. In the upper pole of right kidney and middle part of left kidney, medullary necrosis has only been partial, and there is a central pool of contrast medium seen in the medulla. Precipitating illness was gastroenteritis

infant's electrolytes and hydration were often difficult to manage.

Radiological Findings. Intravenous urograms were carried out between 10 days and 3 weeks after the onset of the kidney lesion. A rapid increase in density of the whole kidney was visible on the first radiograph exposed 5 min after the start of injection. Subsequently this was shown to be a feature of tubular necrosis (Fig. 1a). When tubular necrosis was the dominant lesion the kidney increased in density progressively, often over many hours. In the infants in whom medullary necrosis was the dominant lesion, the medulla became even more heavily opacified within the first 15 min of injection (Fig. 1b). This density was maintained for about $1\frac{1}{2}$ h. During the dense nephrographic phases of tubular and medullary necrosis, contrast medium continued to be cleared into the urine. In an oliguric infant aged 5 days, reported by OGATA et al. [12] no evidence of function was seen at intravenous urography (IVU) although an aortogram showed an abnormal nephrographic phase.

3.2. Late Studies

Gradually the excessive water and solute loss seen in the polyuric phase abated. Follow-up studies carried out after 3 months and more have shown a return to a normal urographic appearance when there has been previous evidence of tubular necrosis.

When medullary necrosis was the dominant lesion, the kidney frequently showed varying degrees of residual medullary damage: caliectasis followed the total loss of medullary tissue, and pools of contrast medium in a medulla were seen when medullary loss was subtotal (Fig. 2). Similar findings have been reported by NOGRADY and LESK [11]. Widespread caliectasis could be mistaken for pyelonephritic scarring in later life. Until recently, severe medullary damage had been found at follow-up, but in the last 18 months one case has been encountered where there were normal urographic findings at follow-up (Fig. 1c). It would seem likely that, if there is no thrombosis in the vasa recta of the medulla, recovery of the parenchymal cells can occur.

3.3. Experimental Confirmation of the Urographic Findings

The need for an experimental study became apparent during the course of the illness in the first case encountered (radiograph shown in Figure 2). Because the nature of the kidney lesion was a matter for conjecture at the time, open renal biopsy was carried out: only cortex was studied, and this showed that tubular necrosis was present. Yet the greatest density was seen in the medulla, and this needed to be explained. Accordingly, experimental studies of the urographic appearances in the rat with tubular necrosis and medullary necrosis were undertaken.

Acute Tubular Necrosis. Rats were given mercury chloride, which induced tubular necrosis. Subsequent urography showed a rapidly developing nephrogram of uniformly increased and protracted density [14]. This study confirmed findings made earlier by CHAMBERLAIN and SHERWOOD [3].

Medullary Necrosis. Rats were given ethylinamine, which induced medullary necrosis. Subsequent urography [14] showed an exceptionally dense opacification of the medulla, thus confirming the idea that the dense medullary opacification in the infant was a feature of medullary necrosis.

The reason why the renal parenchyma is exceptionally dense when there is cell damage can be explained on the basis of the work of BANK et al. [1]. In their study of tubular necrosis in rats, they showed that the fate of the dye lissamine green could be traced by photomicrographs. After an intravenous injection, the dye was cleared through the glomerulus and into the lumen of the nephron. In the normal kidney the dye remained in the lumen. When there was tubular necrosis, the dye passed into the nephron, but subsequently it leaked from the lumen of the nephron into the interstitial spaces.

This explanation can be applied to the urographic findings. The contrast medium sodium diatrizoate (Hypaque) is dealt with by the kidney in the same way as lissamine green. Leakage of contrast medium into the interstitial tissues of the kidney would certainly make the kidney image denser, as the number of iodine atoms inside the nephron and in the interstitial tissues increased. Such leakage could also account for the rapid increase in density of the kidney image in tubular and medullary necrosis, for Bank and co-workers showed that lissamine green leakage occurred within seconds of the intravenous injection of the dye. It is conceivable that, as cells are lost during parenchymal necrosis, sodium diatrizoate could also accumulate in larger quantities in their place.

In former times there was a conflict between those who said that in tubular necrosis there was obstruction of nephrons and those who said there must be leakage from the nephrons [10]. The evidence from these more recent experimental studies and the radiological findings all point to the importance of leakage when there is kidney cell necrosis; a point made by RICHARDS in 1929 [13].

4. Clinical Features and Radiological Findings in Renal Venous Thrombosis

4.1. Clinical Features

It is difficult to find any really significant distinction between the primary illnesses leading to tubular and medullary necrosis and those leading to renal venous thrombosis. Many studies have emphasized that gastroenteritis is a common precursor of renal venous thrombosis. The shock state appears to be common to all.

The infant who develops renal venous thrombosis characteristically has a large kidney on palpation and haematuria. One or both kidneys may be affected. Quite rapidly the renal mass becomes smaller and the haematuria abates. The veno-occlusive lesion is thought to start in small-renal veins and progress to the larger renal vein.

4.2. Radiological Findings

At intravenous urography, if contrast medium is injected into a vein of the lower limb, a cavogram may show no blood entering the vena cava from the affected kidney. Extension of clot into the lumen of the vena cava from the renal vein may be evident, especially on lateral radiographic projection [8].

In the excretion phase of the urogram, the kidney which is the site of recent renal venous thrombosis shows no clearance of contrast medium: that is, there is no nephrogram and no calyx opacification (Fig. 3a). At this time the normal structure of the collecting system is maintained (Fig. 3b). Follow-up studies after a short period of time (say, 3 weeks) can show the kidney size has dimin-

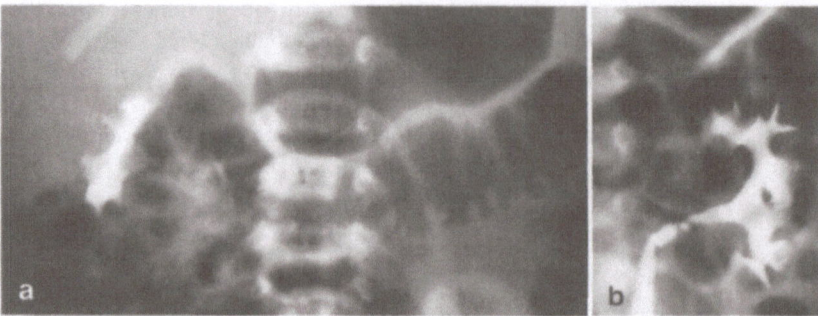

Fig. 3a and b. a) Renal venous thrombosis is associated with a left renal mass which shows no function at IVU in the acute phase Infant born by breech delivery: mother was a diabetic

b) Retrograde study shows intact calyx system during the acute phase. Subsequently this kidney became very small, with clubbed calyces, and it showed poor function at IVU

ished rapidly, and the small kidney has clubbed calyces. In these circumstances there has been a major degree of irreversible parenchymal damage. This is not always the sequence in renal venous thrombosis. Recovery of function in a kidney of apparently normal structure may be seen (Fig. 4). When this happens, it must be surmised that renal venous occlusion has affected only small veins, and that recanalization has occurred.

5. Involvement of other Organs in the Shock State

Cerebral damage is a well-recognised sequel to hypoxia and shock in the neonate. There is evidence to suggest that this is associated with a consumptive coagulopathy [2]. One infant who had kidney damage (tubular and medullary necrosis)

is showing signs of mental retardation as he grows older.

In a large series of patients with adrenal haemorrhagic necrosis EKLÖF and coworkers found that neonatal hypoxia had been a common antecedant [6]. It is thought that adrenal haemorrhagic necrosis is a result of severe stress, and that as its consequence there is adrenal overactivity [9]. One child who had features of bilateral renal venous thrombosis had no function at IVU in the first urogram: follow-up urography showed a calcifying adrenal haemorrhage (Fig. 4).

6. Conclusion

Study of medullary necrosis, tubular necrosis and renal venous thrombosis shows that, although there is an exceptionally wide range of clinical

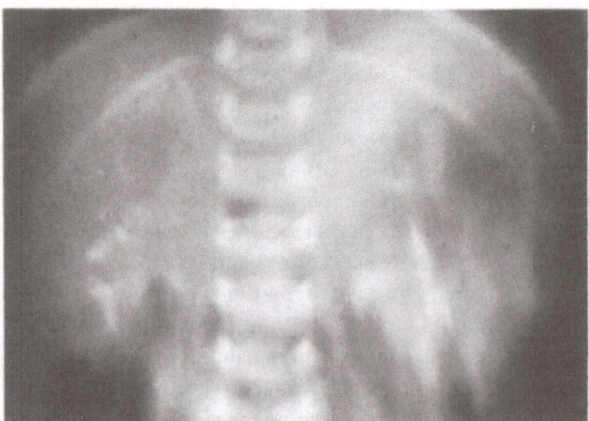

Fig. 4. This infant had no evidence of kidney function at IVU during a phase when the kidneys were palpable and haematuria was present. IVU 3 weeks later shows left kidney is normal. Right kidney is rather small, and there is a calcifying adrenal haematoma above right kidney (tomogram). It has been inferred that right kidney has been the site of renal venous thrombosis, and that recovery of this kidney has occurred. Precipitating illness: infection with diarrhoea and vomiting

antecedants, all of these have the shock state in common. This leads to kidney injury which may be transient. When renal venous thrombosis and medullary necrosis have occurred, the kidney may sustain permanent damage. Radiology provides techniques uniquely appropriate to the study of these forms of kidney injury.

References

1. BANK, N., MUTZ, B. F., AYNEDIJIAN, H. S.: The role of "leakage" of tubular fluid in anuria due to mercury poisoning. J. Clin. Invest. **46**, 695 (1967)
2. CHADD, M. A., ELWOOD, P. C., MUXWORTHY, S. M.: Coagulation defects in hypoxic full-term new born infants. Br. med. J. **IV**, 516 (1971)
3. CHAMBERLAIN, M. J., SHERWOOD, T.: Intravenous urography in experimental acute renal failure in the rat Nephron **4**, 65 (1967)
4. CHRISPIN, A. R., HULL, D., LILLIE, J. G., RISDON, R. A.: Renal tubular necrosis and papillary necrosis after gastroenteritis in infants. Br. med. J. **1**, 410 (1970)
5. CHRISPIN, A. R.: Medullary necrosis in infancy. British Medical Bulletin **28**, 233 (1972)
6. EKLÖF, O., GROTTE, G., JORULF, H., LÖHR, G., RINGERTZ, H.: Perinatal haemorrhagic necrosis of the adrenal gland: a clinical and radiological evaluation of 24 consecutive cases. Pediat. Radiol. **4**, 31 (1975)
7. HEENE, D. L.: In: Microcirculation, Haemostasis and Shock, pp. 103—109. Stuttgart: Schattauer, 1970
8. KNAPP, K.: In: Proceedings: XIII International Congress of Pediatrics, Vol. XIV: Malignant Diseases, Radiology and Nuclear Medicine, p. 301. Wien: Wiener Medizinische Akademie 1971
9. MARGARETTEN, W.: In: Microcirculation, Haemostasis and Shock, p. 125. Stuttgart: Schattauer 1970
10. MERRILL, J. P.: In: Diseases of the Kidney. STRAUSS, M. B., WELT, L. G. (eds.), p. 646. Boston: Little Brown and Co. 1971
11. NOGRADY, M. B., LESK, D. M.: Renal papillary necrosis in the newborn. A case report with roentgenologic documentation of late sequelae. Amer. J. Roentgenol. **116** 661 (1972)
12. OGATA, E. S., GOODING, C. A., PHIBBS, R. H.: Angiographic and ultrasonic appearance of renal cortical necrosis in the newborn. Pediat. Radiol. **3**, 226 (1975)
13. RICHARDS, A. N.: Trans. Ass. Am. Physns. **44**, 64 (1929)
14. RISDON, R. A., BERRY, C. L., CHRISPIN, A. R.: Urographic changes in acute papillary necrosis in the rat. Br. med. J. **III**, 263 (1970)

The Radiology of the Vesico-Ureteric Junction

H. Fendel

The main factors causing urinary tract disease are: infection, obstruction, reflux, and renal calculi. These four horsemen of the apocalypse cooperate like a modern martial commando unit (Fig. 1). Each horseman rarely appears alone, and each is prepared to shoot the road free for any of the others or for the whole group, or provide a fire-shield for a particular one when attacked. Obstruction and reflux may lead to infection and stone formation, stones may cause infection or obstruction, infection may precede stones, produce obstructive lesions, or damage those structures which normally protect against reflux. The horseman on the right wing of the cavalcade represents urinary calculi. He looks somewhat older, and he is a little less important, although not insignificant in children. The one in the center obviously is in the prime of his life. He represents

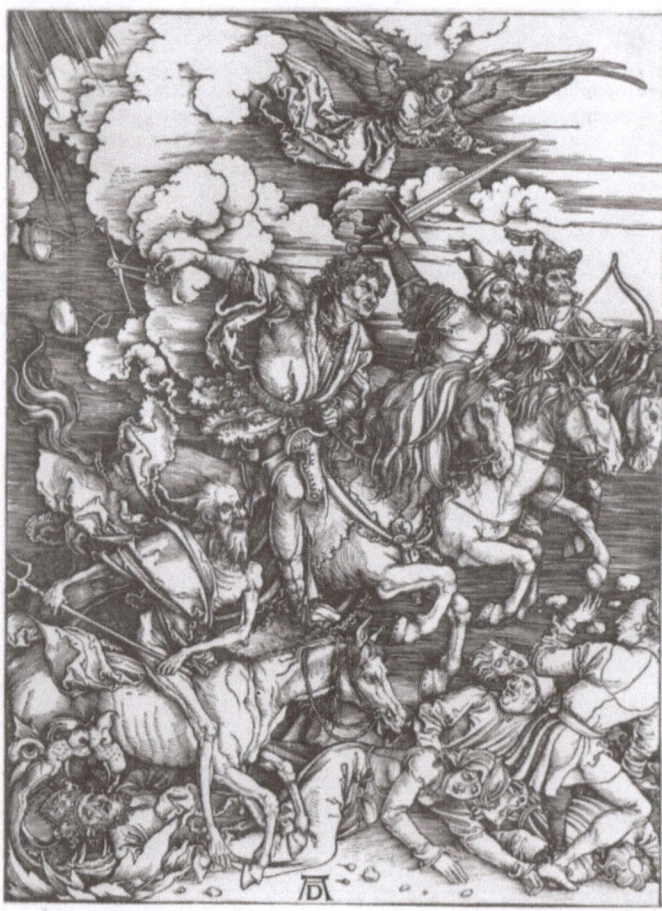

Fig. 1. The four horsemen of the apocalypse. Woodcut by ALBRECHT DÜRER. Courtesy of Staatliche Graphische Sammlung München

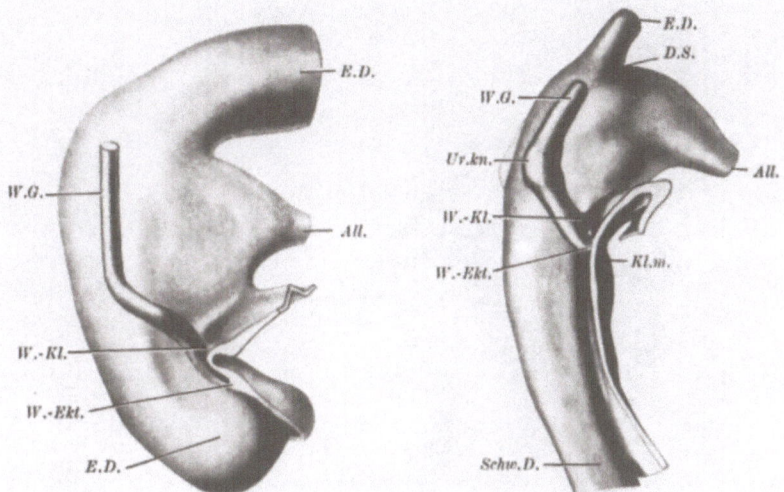

Fig. 2. CHWALLA's model of the caudal part of an embryo of 3.4 mm (left) and 4.8 mm (right) length. W.G. = Wolffian duct. E.D. = hind gut. All. = Allantois. W.-Kl. = junction between Wolffian duct and cloaca. W.-Ekt. = junction between Wolffian duct and ectoderm. Kl.m. = cloacal membrane. Ur.kn. = ureteral bud. (Reproduced from VON HAYEK [4]

infection and apparently is the true leader of the group. The left wing looks remarkably strong and dangerous. Here two horsemen ride side by side, one representing obstruction, the other reflux. They look very similar, like brothers or even twins, and, in fact, obstruction and reflux may have deleterious effects on the urinary tract which are very similar. Both of them impede the transport of urine with the potential risk of overload and backpressure. Both of them free the way for infection, obstruction by urinary stasis, reflux by the yo-yoing to and fro of the urinary stream, and, reflux in addition by transporting bacteria up to and into the kidney.

I do not know exactly the meaning of the *angel* hovering over the scene. Perhaps, it is merely an orthographic characteristic since I am going to discuss the vesico-ureteric junction and the *angle* which is formed where the ureter enters the bladder wall. Let us assume it to be a guardian-angel against the dangerous group. Continuing with this analogy it is the spirit of pediatric radiology which provides the crucial information in these cases and pediatric radiology is now in the scenario.

Junctions between sections of tube-like organs are usually the most critical points for either obstruc-

tion or backflow. The normal and abnormal conditions which exist or can exist at these particular points can neither be understood nor assessed without appreciation of the anatomy and function of the region concerned. At the vesicoureteric junction, the interweaving of structures is very complicated, and no clear understanding of the interesting features can be reached without looking at the course of embryological events which take place here in very early human life.

At the 4 mm stage (Fig. 2), that is in the 4th week of gestation, the primitive endodermal cloaca is undivided. The Wolffian ducts, which are the mesonephric collecting tubes, arise near the anterior part of the cloacal membrane. Between the 4 mm and 6 mm stage, that is between the 4th and 6th weeks of gestation, a subdivision of the primitive cloaca takes place by downward growth of the urorectal septum as far as Müller's hillock (which is the verumontanum) and by lateral ingrowths of the mesenchyme caudal to this level. At the same time, the Wolffian ducts recede to the level of the verumontanum where the terminal segments of the Wolffian ducts now open into the cloaca as the common excretory ducts. Simultaneously, somewhat craniolateral to these openings, the ureteral buds appear as outgrowths of the Wolffian

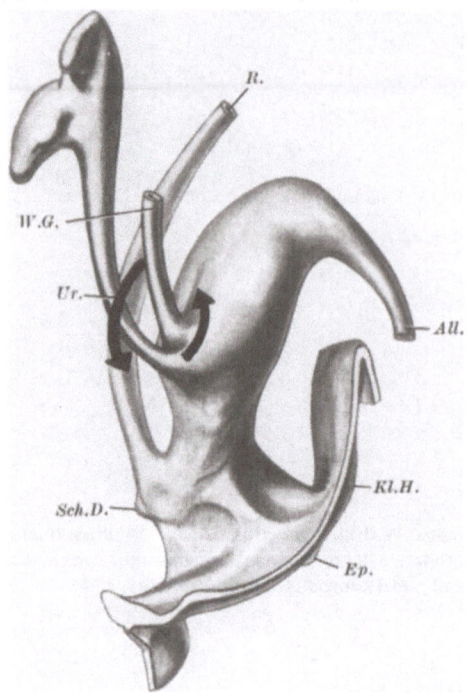

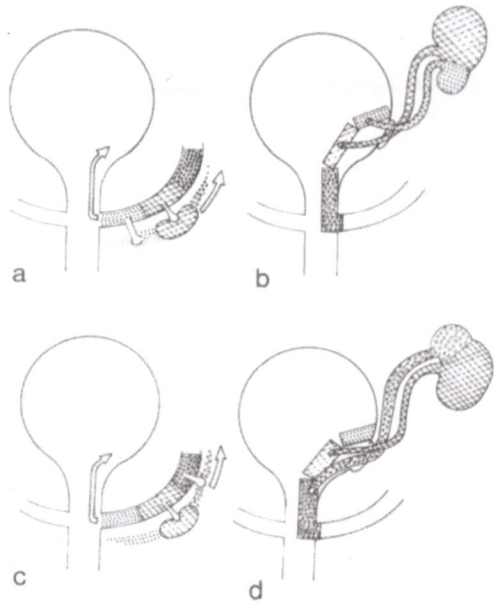

Fig. 4. The relationship of the primary and final position of the mesodermal zones of the distal Wolffian duct, the final position of the ureteric orifices, the original position of the ureteric buds, and the location of the nephrogenic blastema in cases of duplicated ureters before (a and c) and after (b and d) migration. The distal part of the Wolffian duct comes to the interiordorsal side of the primitive vesico-urinary canal. In this way, mesodermal material builds up the superficial trigone down to the verumontanum in the male, down the external urethral meatus in the female. The caudal zone of the distal Wolffian duct forms the cranio-lateral part of the superficial trigone, the middle zone its caudal-medial part, and the cranial zone the superficial structures of the bladder neck and posterior urethra. A supernumerary ureteric outgrowth of the caudal zone (a) is finally placed in a cranio-laterally dystopic position (b), a supernumerary ureteric bud of the cranial zone (c) finally opens in a caudo-medially dystopic or ectopic position (d). The accessory buds do not always strike the nephrogenic blastema in a sufficient manner. Consequently, the more the position of the accessory bud deviates from that of the normal one, the more the accessory kidney segment is prone to be finally dysplastic. In case a a caudal dysplastic kidney segment results from a caudal accessory bud, in case c a cranial dysplastic moiety from a cranial one. (Theory and figure from G. G. MACKIE and F. D. STEPHENS [6])

Fig. 3. CHWALLA's model of the caudal part of an embryo of 10.3 mm length. R. = rectum All. = allantois. W.G. = Wolffian duct Ur. = ureter. (Reproduced from VON HAYEK [4]). The arrows demonstrate the twisting migration of the primitive ureter and the WOLFFIAN duct

ducts, and they push dorsocranially into the blastema of the primordial kidneys. The common excretory ducts, together with a small segment of the Wolffian ducts cranial to the ureteral buds, are then included in the formation of the vesicourinary canal (Fig. 3). By a peculiar, twisting mediocranial migration these mesodermal structures come to lie on the interior and dorsal side of the vesicourinary canal, and, they build up the crista urethralis, the superficial trigone with Bell's muscle and the intravesical ureteric segment, and the whole ureter.

The twisting upward migration of the mesodermal derivatives is responsible for the so-called Weigert-Meyer rule, namely, that (with very few exceptions) in cases of duplication of the ureter the orifice of the ureter draining the upper renal segment lies more or less caudo medial to the one draining the lower renal segment, and so the extravesical ureters cross one another (Fig. 4).

The endodermal derivatives, namely, urethra, deep trigone, and Waldeyer's sheath on the one hand, and the mesodermal derivatives, namely, crista urethralis, superficial trigone, and intravesical ureter on the other, remain distinct entities. The superficial trigone lies on the deep trigone. Both are delicately connected, but easy to separate by dissection. Their nerve supply is different, and their motions during bladder distention and contraction are to a certain degree free, one against the other. More caudally the distal parts of the superficial trigone and the crista urethralis become more and more attached to the deeper structures and in this way the ureters and the superficial trigone are anchored at the point from which they originated (Fig. 5).

A second effective, but nevertheless comparably loose, fixation exists at the two upper cornua of the trigone where the intramural segment of the ureters are surrounded by the delicate collagen and elastic fibers of Waldeyer's sheath. The ureteric orifice lies in the trigone. The orifice is in no respect an end-point of a tube. It is only the end of the lumen of the ureter, but all the ureteric structures continue within the network of the superficial trigone, being essentially an indivisible part of it.

In the course of the aforementioned embryological events, some deviations can occur. We have already mentioned the double anlage of the ure-

teral bud by way of which a *ureter duplex* develops. This must clearly be differentiated from the splitting of a primary single bud, the result of which is a *ureter fissus*. The ultimate point of bi-

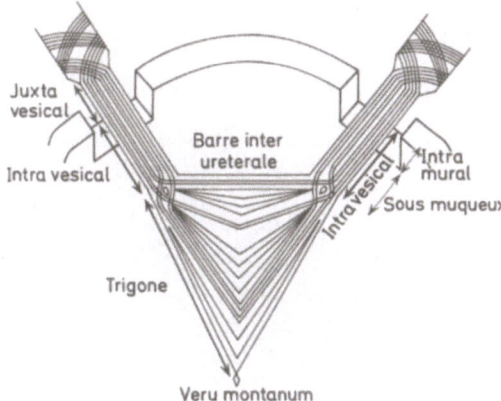

Fig. 5. Schematic drawing of the uretero-trigonal musculature. (Drawing from GRÉGOIR, W., DEBLED, G. [3].) Just prevesically the spiral muscle fibers of the ureter change to a completely longitudinal orientation. At the point of the ureteric orifice the ureteral structures lose their lumen but continue as the superficial trigone down to the point they originated from: the verumontanum in the male and the external urethral meatus in the female

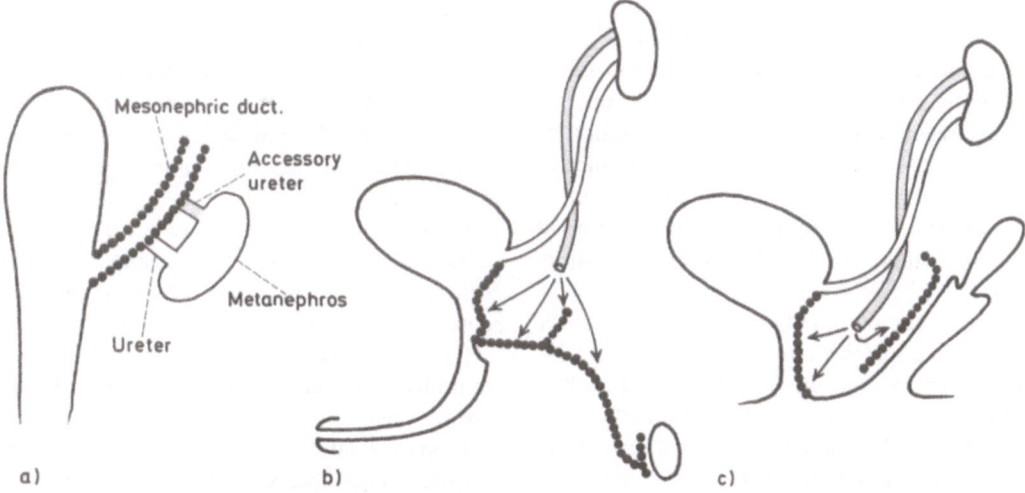

Fig. 6. a) An *ectopic* accessory ureter always drains the upper segment of a duplex kidney, and both result from a cranial accessory primitive ureteral outgrowth. The accessory ureteric orifice follows the migration of the mesodermal material of the Wolffian duct. b) The possible sites of an *ectopic* ureteral opening in the male are: the bladder neck, the posterior urethra as low as

the verumontanum, the ejaculatory duct, the seminal vesicle, the vas deferens, and—at least theoretically—the epididymal canal. c) In the female: the bladder neck, the dorsal wall of the whole urethra, the vulva adjacent to the urethral meatus, or the Gärtner's duct. (Drawings from JOHNSTON, J. H. [5].)

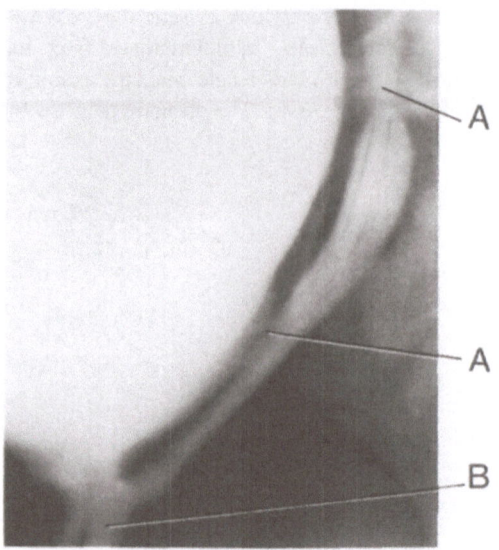

Fig. 7. Duplication of the left kidney and ureter in a 7-year-old girl. Both ureteral openings are incompetent. A) Vesico-ureteric reflux into the lower renal segment; slight weakness of the trigone but sufficient length and angle of the cranial uretero-vesical junction. B) Ectopic opening of the cranial ureter in the dorsal wall of the distal urethra. The cranial moiety of the kidney and the cranial ureter except its distal segment have been removed 3 years ago. The urethro-ureteral reflux into the blind loop must be considered the source of frequent ascending infections in this girl

furcation can be located at any level of the ureter, within the renal pelvis, the extravesical upper or lower ureter, prevesically, or in its intramural or submucosal segment. The clinical significance of the particular levels of the bifurcation varies so that in cases of renal duplication the radiological diagnostic approach should encompass this question.

The openings of completely duplicated ureters can lie close together at the normal place or at a greater or smaller distance from each other. Usually both are not at the right place, the position of one being more craniolateral, that of the other more caudomedial. In many cases the ureter of the cranial renal segment drains into the bladder outlet or ectopically to the bladder (Fig. 6). Ectopic ureters in the male can open into the posterior urethra, the ejaculatory duct, the seminal vesicle, the vas deferens or the epididymal canal, all of which are derivatives of the Wolffian duct.

In the female the ectopic orifice can be located in the posterior wall of the urethra, in the introitus vaginae adjacent to the external urethral meatus, or it may drain via Gärtner's duct into the vagina, very rarely into the uterus itself (Fig. 7). In both sexes, the ectopic ureter can also drain into the rectum, but this aberration is extremely rare and usually associated with severe and complex malformations of the rectum and anus.

Ectopic ureters can develop cyst-like dilatations of their submucosal segment which protrude into the bladder cavity and/or the urethra. Dynamically these ectopic ureteroceles cause obstruction of their ureters, and, in addition, they can obstruct the ipsilateral and/or contralateral orifice and/or the bladder outlet and urethra. The protruding ureterocoele can rupture so that it becomes smaller or even seems to disappear. In this way and in addition to the ectopic orifice, one or more accessory openings develop which may be called uretero-vesical fistulae or—the larger ones—uretero-vesical windows (Figs. 8a, b, c).

Figure 9a shows the findings in a 5 month old female infant with a right sided ectopic ureterocele which has a small additional opening in its right lower part. In the 10 year old girl of Figure 9c the ureterocele was no longer prominent presumably because of rupture in its upper half where there is now a larger uretero-vesical window. In a 7 year old girls whose findings are demonstrated in Figure 9b the ectopic ureterocele could no longer be seen, but two large windows were found to have developed in the course of the preceding protrusion.

Ureteroceles of single ureters are less frequent in children than in adults, but these simple ureteroceles do occur in the paediatric age range and should not be overlooked (Fig. 10). A much less frequent finding is a so-called everted ureterocele; the protruding segment of the ureter on occasion slips through the ureteric hiatus of the bladder wall and evaginates.

Dystopia and ectopia of a single ureter follows the rules previously set out in respect of a supernumerary ureter. With very few exceptions the dystopic or ectopic opening lies anywhere on the line given by the embryologic migration of the primitive ureteral orifice. It follows from what we learned from embryology that a caudo-medially

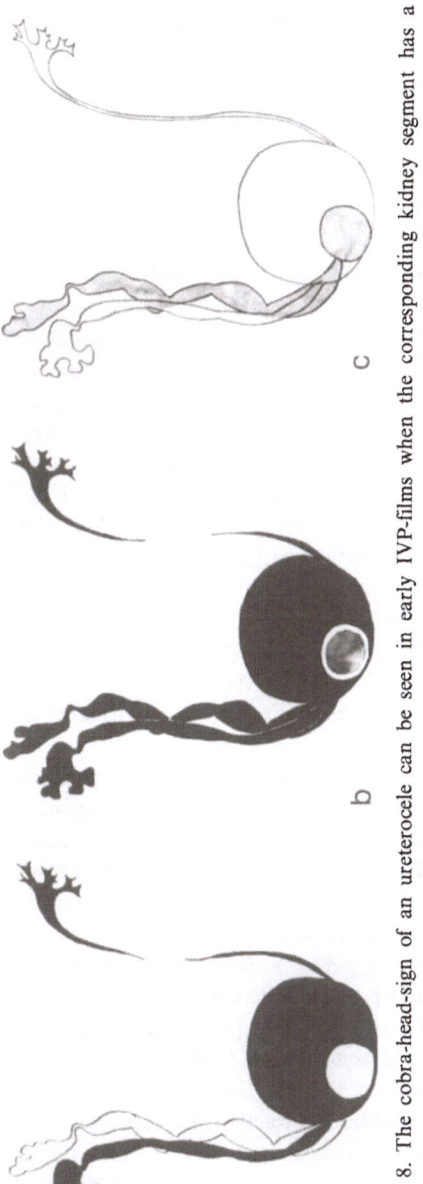

Fig. 8. The cobra-head-sign of an ureterocele can be seen in early IVP-films when the corresponding kidney segment has a reduced excretory function (a) (a) when both kidney segments excrete equally (b) the cobra-head-sign can be demonstrated after evacuation of the bladder (c). (Drawings from FLACH, A., MILDENBERGER, H., FENDEL, H. [2])

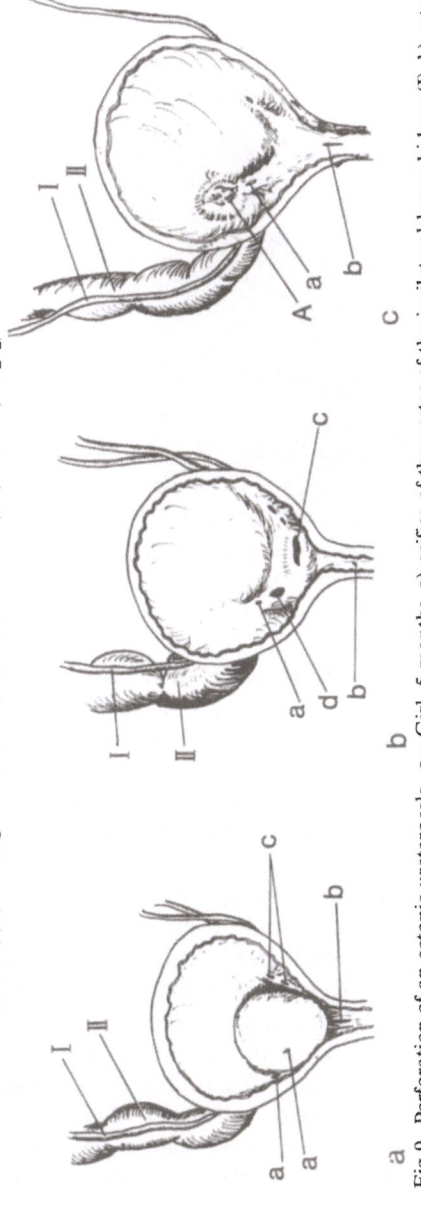

Fig. 9. Perforation of an ectopic ureterocele. a = Girl, 5 months. a) orifice of the ureter of the ipsilateral lower kidney (I), b) ectopic opening of the ureter of the ipsilateral upper renal segment. c) openings of the contralateral duplex ureters. d) small additional opening of the ureterocele which is still existing. b = Girl, 7 years. a) opening of the ureter of the lower kidney segment (I). b) ectopic opening of the ureter of the cranial kidney segment (II). c) and d) two additional openings from the ureterocele which protrudes only slightly. c = Girl, 10 years. a) opening of the ureter of the lower kidney segment (I). b) ectopic opening of the ureter of the cranial renal segment (II). A = large uretero-vesical window after perforation of an ureterocele which is no longer visible. (From MILDENBERGER, H., FENDEL, H., FLACH, A. [8])

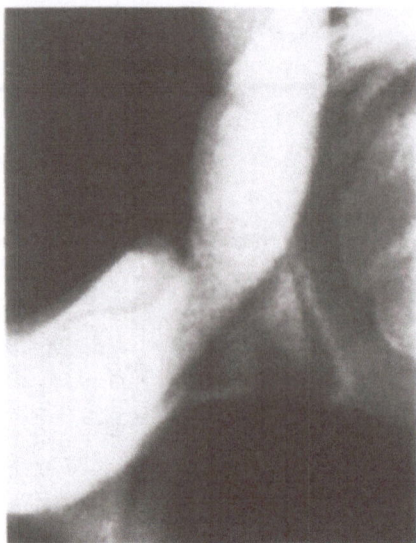

Fig. 10. Small ureterocele without renal duplication (simplex-type) in a 6-year-old boy

dystopic single ureteral opening must be associated with a trigonal hypoplasia, and an ectopic single one with a complete aplasia of the ipsilateral hemitrigone.

Unlike other tube-like organs, the ureter does not possess a double layer of muscle, a circular and a longitudinal one. The ureteral musculature consists of only one layer of crossing spirals of muscle bundles. Just prevesically, this helix-like orientation of the ureteral muscle fibers changes completely into a strictly longitudinal arrangement of the muscularis of the intramural and submucosal segment. This feature enables the normal passage of urine, impelled by the peristaltic activity of the prevesical ureter. The intravesical ureter is not capable of peristalsis. Nevertheless it is not a passive tube. Contraction of its muscle fibers shortens its length without reducing the caliber of its lumen and opens the ureteral orifice.

The ureteral musculature develops comparably late. Until the second month of gestation the ureters are devoid of muscle. It takes a long period of foetal life—from the 2nd to the 6th month—for the ureters to acquire a definitive muscular coat, and the distal segment is the last portion to acquire muscle. For some reasons, as yet not well understood, the characteristic transition of the

muscle arrangement at the uretero-vesical junction can be abnormal in differing degrees and in differing ways (Fig. 11). The muscle bundles can be predominantly circular, while longitudinal fibers are sparse or almost completely absent (abnormal orientation). The number of muscle fibers can be abnormally low and the mass of collagen tissue comparably large. Smooth muscle bundles can appear to be pulled apart by the fibrotic tissue, be thin, or interrupted, or asymmetrically oriented around the lumen. Apparently the severest degree of this fibro-muscular dysplasia of the uretero-vesical junction consists of a completely fibrotic ureteral circumference. This fibro-muscular dysplasia is by no means a true stenosis. To some degree the same appearance can arise in long-standing intramural inflammation. However, this fibro-muscular dysplasia has nothing to do with a stenotic stricture. Nevertheless it is functionally obstructive (Fig. 12).

There is the concept of the so-called congenital or primary megaloureter. In this there is no obstruction, no vesico-ureteric reflux, no abnormality of bladder, trigone or ureteric orifice, and there is no obstruction to vesical outflow. This concept needs revision. The terminal and intramural segment can be the site of achalasia and there may be associated reflux: these features result from an intrinsic developmental error and they often coincide with trigonal dysplasia.

Vesico-ureteric reflux is normally prevented by distinctive trigonal characteristics. First, the ureteral orifice is an integral part of the superficial trigone, and this is attached to the deep structures of the posterior urethra. During bladder distension and bladder contraction the superficial trigone actively stretches itself, and the orifice and lumen of the intravesical ureter is closed: this closure effectively prevents backflow, although an orthograde jet-stream of urine can be pushed out intermittently. Second, the lumen of the submucosal ureteral segment is passively compressed by the rising bladder pressure: this mechanism is less effective when the submucosal tunnel is short. Third, the intramural segment passes obliquely through the bladder wall. The more the bladder is filled, the more acute becomes the angle between the lumen of the bladder and the intramural segment.

Normal

Abnormal Orientation

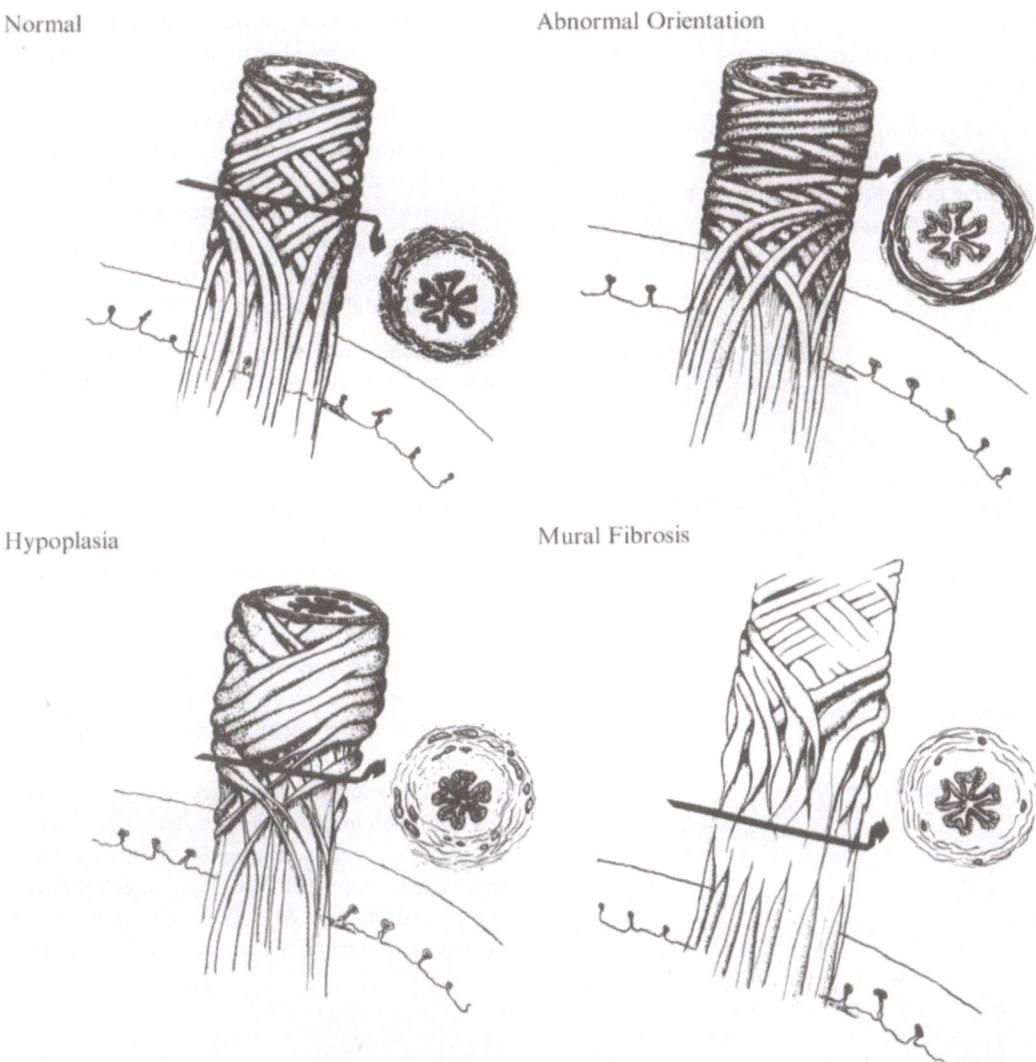

Hypoplasia

Mural Fibrosis

Fig. 11. Schematic drawing of the normal and three different types of abnormal orientation of ureteral smooth muscle bundles at the uretero-vesical junction. *Normal:* the oblique bundles of the prevesical ureter undergo transition into longitudinal arrangement in the intramural ureter. *Abnormal orientation:* The arrangement of the prevesical muscle bundles is more or purely circular with abrupt transition in longitudinal orientation. Closed circular bundles do not elongate correctly, and produce sphincteric obstruction. *Hypo-* *plasia:* In this type, muscle bundles are widely seperated and attenuated, breaks of muscle fibers are obvious and the amount of collagen fibers is increased. The prevesical and intramural ureteral segment is more or less adynamic. *Mural fibrosis:* Only isolated smooth muscle bundles can be seen within a predominant number of collagen fibers. The abundance of collagen restricts ureteral distensibility and limits urine flow. (Findings and drawings by McLAUGHLIN, A.P.)

When there is a vesico-ureteric reflux, these characteristics change to a greater or lesser degree. The orifice is displaced to the cranio-lateral cornu of the trigone. The submucosal segment is short, or is completely absent (Fig. 13a, b). Depending on the degree of shortening of the submucosal segment and on the extent of lateral displacement, the appearance of the orifice changes. When the intramural segment is short and at right-angles to the vesical contour or when this segment is displaced outside the bladder the highest degree of incompetence can be anticipated for the last barrier against reflux has been breached (Fig. 13c).

Obviously the appearance and position of the ureteral orifice can be investigated by cystoscopy. By the same procedure the length of the submucosal tunnel can be ascertained by the use of small

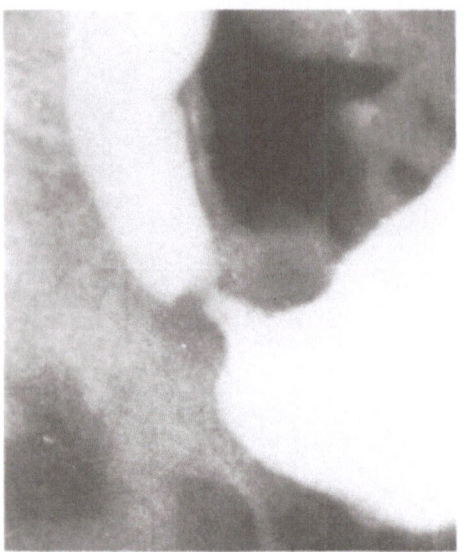

Fig. 12. Distal ureteral achalasia due to fibro-muscular dysplasia of the uretero-vesical junction. Refilling of the bladder after gross vesico-ureteric reflux

probes. The best and now most widely used classification of the endoscopic findings was introduced by Lyon, Marshall and Tanagho. They grade the position of the orifice in grades A to C, the normal being position A, and the most lateral C. When there is first degree shortening of the tunnel and first degree lateral displacement, the small normal peak of intrusion of the normal ureteral opening is cut off: it then looks like a crater or a stadium with the ureteral opening in its cranio-lateral wall.

In the second stage, the caudo-medial wall of the stadium is lost and the ureteral opening then lies flat against its background: the orifice then looks like a horseshoe. In the third grade, the orifice gapes like a golf-hole, and there is no tunnel at all. The submucosal segment and the orifice itself lie beyond the scope of radiology. On the other hand, the intramural ureteral segment usually lies beyond the reach of cystoscopy. Only in those grossly abnormal cases, where there is a gaping golf-hole orifice, can the intramural segment be seen at endoscopy. However, the intramural segment can be clearly demonstrated radiologically. It follows that in order to obtain full information about the uretero-vesical junction the investigatory approach must be by both radiology and endoscopy. The endoscopic and radiological findings must be put together to reach a comprehensive evaluation (Figs. 14a, b). As yet, we have not encountered normal endoscopic findings in con-

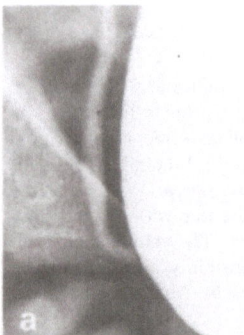
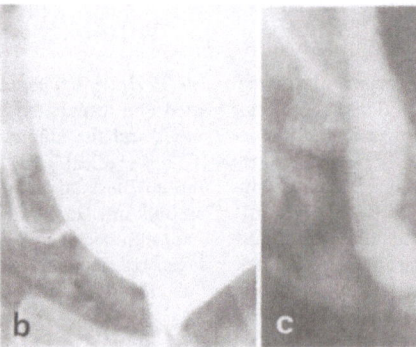

Fig. 13. Incompetence of the vesico-ureteric junction. The abnormality includes the intramural segment which is the last barrier against reflux. This radiologic diagnosis ("Ureterfehleinmündung") implies that with very few exceptions the vesico-ureteral reflux will persist for many years. a) The intramural segment is short and the angle of the junction is more than 45° degrees.

b) Fish-hook-appearance with a right-angled and short intramural segment. a and b are findings in newborn babies without any foregoing urinary tract infection. c) Gross incompetence of the uretero-vesical junction. After a 4 years history of recurrent urinary tract infection the right-angled intramural segment gapes and free reflux occurs

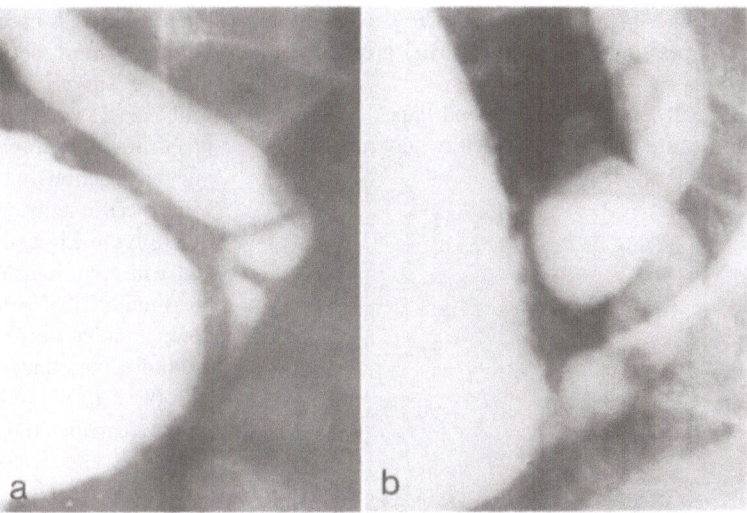

Fig. 14 a and b. Two similar but different findings at the uretero-vesical junction. a) Distal ureteral dynamic stenosis due to fibro-muscular dysplasia but normal length and angle of the intramural segment. b) Abnor- mal intramural segment and pig-tail-appearance of the distal ureter due to widening and lenghtening of the ureter by long standing reflux disease

junction with the radiological finding of a short right-angle intramural segment. On the other hand we have seen normal intramural segments at radiology in cases where the endoscopic findings were abnormal. In our 10 years experience we have seen no single case in which the radiological finding of a short right-angled intramural segment returned to normal. With only very few exceptions, reflux neither improved nor disappeared in these cases. According to the literature, however, reflux can improve or disappear under conservative treatment even though the orifice is in the B or C position and it has either grade 1 or 2, or even 3 appearance at endoscopy.

The consequences of gross vesico-ureteric reflux are: first, quasi-obstruction by the direct transmission of the high intravesical pressure up to the renal pelvis and by backflow overload, and second, upward spread of common infections from the lower urinary tract up to the renal pelvis and into the renal parenchyma (Fig. 15). The last barrier against ascending pyelonephritis is at the tip of the renal papillae. As it was shown first in animal experiments, this barrier can be defective mainly in the upper or lower pole of the kidney so that during high pressure reflux a pelvi-renal influx occurs, causing a segmental ascending paren-

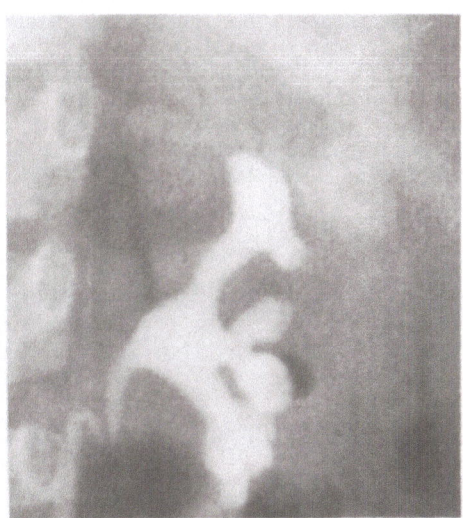

Fig. 15. Pelvi-renal reflux (influx) in a 1½-year-old girl after the first urinary tract infection

chymal inflammation which is followed by gross scarring. Hence, gross vesico-ureteral reflux potentially is the promotor of true segmental atrophic pyelonephritis. In addition, the quasi-obstructive effects of gross vesico-ureteral reflux can directly affect renal blood flow and kidney function, and in this way longstanding reflux causes back-pressure atrophy or delayed growth of the kidney as a whole.

Basically, both infection and quasi-obstruction constitute the disease of reflux nephropathy. No

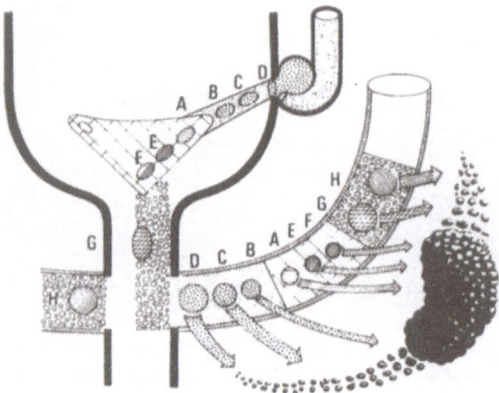

Fig.16. Relationship of the location of the ureteric orifice in bladder and urethra and the points of origin from Wolffian duct. Incompetent ureteral openings displaced cranio-laterally (B, C and D) and associated with a primary uretero-trigonal dysplasia are derivatives from ureteric buds which by their abnormal position induce a focal, segmental or complete renal dysplasia. Thus, the latter is not the result of reflux but a concomitant event. (Theory and drawing by MACKIE, G.G., STEPHENS, F.D. [6])

further debate is necessary: the deleterious course of events must be stopped, in many cases by means of surgery. This does not always solve the problem as a whole and may even give rise to new problems, for example, a transitory or long-standing obstruction at the ureteroneocystostomy which occasionally occurs as a very late complication. But there is no doubt that this operation was and will continue to be of much benefit to the great majority of patients concerned. Meanwhile however, it has been shown in a number of follow-up studies that, under modern diagnostic care and with the help of modern chemotherapy, pyelonephritic scarring and back-pressure atrophy are very rare events in children with mild or moderate vesico-ureteric reflux. In our own experience there was no significant correlation between the presence of moderate reflux and the number of recurrences and the severity or persistence of urinary tract infection. On the other hand, renal size correlated well with the number of recurrences of infection. No significant difference could be found in kidney size in cases with and without reflux, but it was significantly different when one or more consecutive isotope renograms had indicated a transitory pyelonephritis.

Furthermore, not everything which looks like a pyelonephritic scar really is one, and not every

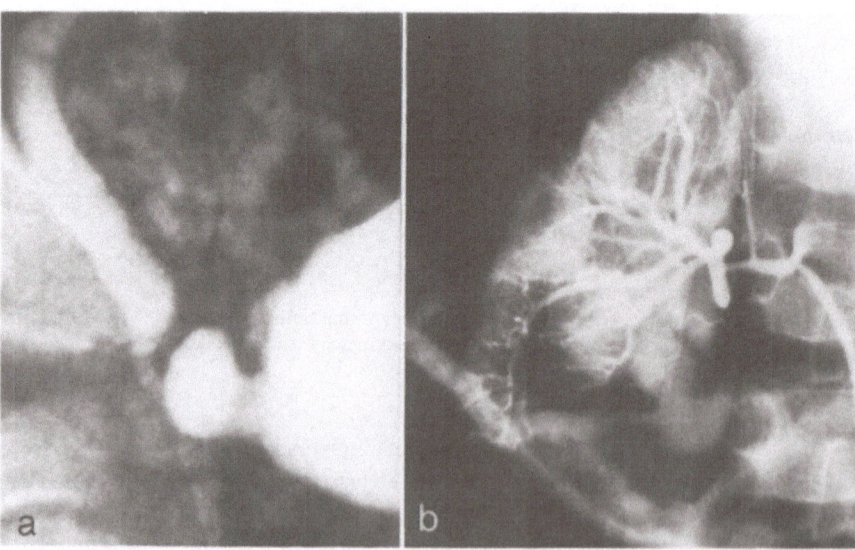

Fig. 17. Extravesicalasation of the ureteral ostium (position D in STEPHENS' schema) associated with a (congenital) small kidney which angiographically shows focal dysplasia predominantly of the lower pole

small kidney is the consequence of reflux transmitted back-pressure. Acquired scarring and severe atrophy can be mimicked by congenital small kidneys or focal renal dysplasia, and these entities obviously are concomitants of trigonal dysplasia and refluxing vesico-ureteric junctions. To understand this we must go back once more to embryology (Fig. 16). The whole story starts at the point of the tiny ureteral bud. When its anlage deviates from the normal point, an abnormal position and a gross or a least microscopic dysplasia of the trigonum results. By the same event it may be that the outgrowth of the primitive ureter does not meet the nephrogenic blastema at the correct location. The association of renal dysplasia with grossly abnormal locations of the ureteral opening is well known. Although it has been somewhat speculative until now, it is the case that even slight aberrations of the ureteral bud can be followed by renal dysplasia involving one pole or the kidney as a whole (Fig. 17). This would explain the fact that even mild reflux is sometimes associated with apparent renal scarring in very young infants who have not had any proven infection. However, parenchymal dysplasia may involve the renal papillae so that the parenchymal barrier is defective and the particular kidney is prone to ascending pyelonephritis when reflux occurs. Thus, the cat bites its own tail, and the vicious circle is completed.

The vesico-ureteric junction is a very small area of the body. Although it is the critical point for many urinary tract anomalies and for a great number of serious urinary tract diseases, it is usually overlooked by many radiologists. Furthermore, the vesico-ureteric junction is far from being as simple as is made out in many articles and textbooks or indeed in many doctors' minds. Safe medical cure depends on an adequate diagnostic approach. Here, indeed, the role of radiology is important.

References

1. CHWALLA, R.: Über die Entwicklung der Harnblase und der primären Harnröhre. Z. Anat. **83**, 616—733 (1927)
2. FLACH, A., MILDENBERGER, H., FENDEL, H.: Ureterozelen im Kindesalter. Med. Welt. **18** (N.F.), 2862—2865 (1967)
3. GRÉGOIR, W., DEBLED, G.: Ätiologie des primären Megaloureters. In LUTZEYER, W., MELCHIOR, H. (Eds.): Ureterdynamik, pp. 24—29, Stuttgart: Thieme Verlag 1972
4. HAYEK, H. v.: Die Entwicklung der Harn- und Geschlechtsorgane. In: ALKEN. C. E., DIX, V. W., GOODWIN, W. E., WILDBOLZ, E. (Eds.): Handbuch der Urologie. Vol. 1 Anatomie und Embryologie, pp. 1—52, Berlin-Heidelberg-New York: Springer-Verlag 1969
5. JOHNSTON, J. H.: Problems in the diagnosis and management of ectopic ureters and ureteroceles. In: JOHNSTON, J. H., SCHOLTMEIJER, R. J. (Eds.): Problems in Paediatric Urology, pp. 57—78, Amsterdam: Excerpta Medica 1972
6. MACKIE, G. G., STEPHENS, F. D.: Duplex kidneys: a correlation of renal dysplasia with position of the ureteral orifice. J. Urol. **114**, 274—280 (1975)
7. MCLAUGHLIN, A. P., PFISTER, R. C., LEADBETTER, W. F., SALZSTEIN, S. L., KESSLER, W. O.: The pathophysiology of primary megaloureter. J. Urol. **109**, 805—811 (1973)
8. MILDENBERGER, H., FENDEL, H., FLACH, A.: Ureterozele im Kindesalter. Bericht über 14 Fälle. Münch. med. Wschr. **110**, 327—332 (1968)

The Prostate in Pediatric Radiology

G. Theander

1. Introduction

The prostate gland in infancy and childhood has received relatively scanty attention either from clinicians and pathologists or from radiologists. The following survey of the various roles played by this organ in pediatric disease is provisional. It is concerned chiefly with radiologic diagnosis, but some anatomical and clinical aspects have been included. Although the topic is limited to the prostate proper, certain intimately connected pathways, such as the prostatic portion of the urethra, must also be considered to some extent. Despite their great importance, obstructing valves and other primarily urethral abnormalities are not described here.

2. Radiologic Examination

Plain radiographs will only rarely demonstrate the prostate in childhood. Even calcification will

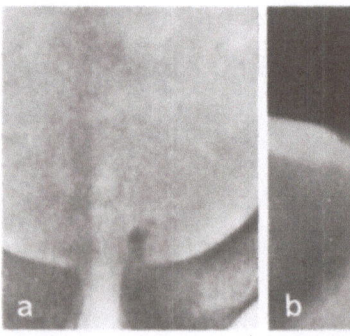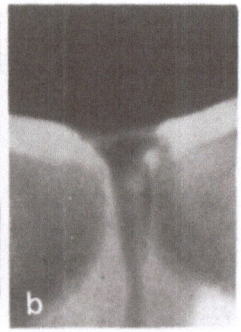

Fig. 1 a and b. Calcification in prostate. 13 years. a) plain film, b) UCG. A-p views. Hemophiliac with long history of urinary infection complicating neurogenic disorder of bladder and paraplegia after hematoma in spinal cord

not provide any clue to the size or shape of the gland, because the calcific deposits are, as a rule, quite small and deep-seated (Fig. 1). Radiologic demonstration of other abnormalities of the gland requires the use of contrast medium.

Although a special procedure has been devised for radiologic examination of the utricle and prostatic ducts [4], it does not seem to have been used in the examination of children. The most informative method has been urethrocystography (UCG), which should include films taken during micturition. However, since prostatic abnormalities frequently reflect a pathologic process or malformation involving the entire urinary system, urography (UG) is also often highly informative. It can hardly be emphasized enough that radiologic exploration of urologic disease in infancy and childhood should comprise both UG and UCG.

3. The Prostatic Tissue

3.1. Malformation

Agenesis of the prostate has been observed as a component of various rare syndromes affecting the development of the hindgut and genito-urinary system. In these grave conditions the lack of the prostate is hardly a feature deserving special attention. In certain other malformations involvement of the prostate is less profound but more important both clinically and radiologically, because such malformations include anomalous channels. These are described below in a separate section.

3.2. Hematoma

Intraprostatic hematoma is a rare condition in newborn infants. It is apt to cause urinary reten-

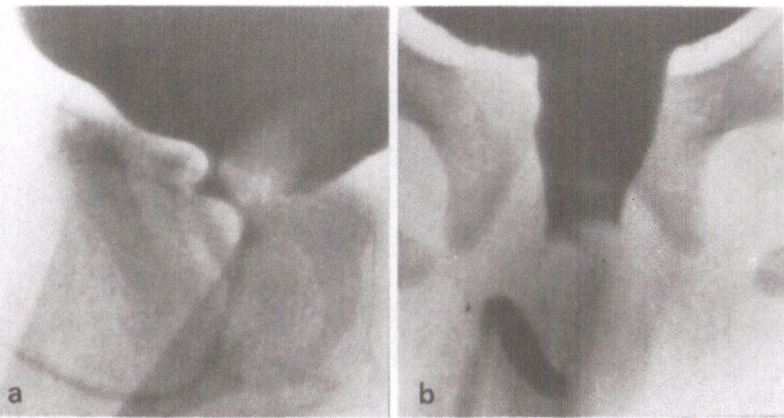

Fig. 2 a and b. Peduncultated polyp at seminal collicle. 1 year. UCG, a) oblique, b) a-p, view. Tip of polyp seen in bladder neck before micturition a), in urethra during micturition b). Catheter in urethra in a). (Courtesy of Dr. OLE EKLÖF)

tion and may become infected. No such case seems to have been diagnosed radiologically.

3.3. Infection

An abscess of the prostate may develop without a pre-existing hematoma. This condition, too, has been clinically recognized in the neonate. Radiologic demonstration of intraprostatic *calcification* of necrotic tissue is evidence of inflammatory disease, which may or may not have healed (Fig. 1). In some cases the deposits represent the walls or contents of cavities communicating with the urethra. Observations made in adults suggest that they are late sequelae to bacterial infection [2]; despite the frequent occurrence of such infection in children prostatic calcifications are rare before puberty. Calcium phosphate *stones* in a prostatic cavity have, however, been radiologically detected in a child as young as 4 years [3].

Infection of the prostate other than abscess is apparently unknown in pediatric pathology, and prominent urologists have claimed that prostatitis does not exist in infancy and childhood. This statement has, however, been challenged by recent observations considered at the end of the present survey.

3.4. Tumours

Benign *polyps* may arise at the verumontanum, i.e., the seminal collicle carrying the openings of several prostatic channels and normally protruding slightly into the posterior wall of the urethra. Such a polyp may become pedunculated and large enough to cause sudden and intermittent obstruction during voiding. Its typical site and mobility are demonstrable at UCG (Fig. 2). Since the polyps actually belong to the urethral mucosa rather than to the prostate proper, they may also originate in other parts of the urethral wall.

All *true neoplasms* of the prostate before puberty appear to be malignant. They are practically always embryonic rhabdomyosarcomas. Prostatic leiomyosarcoma, angiosarcoma and carcinoma do exist in childhood, but they are extremely rare. A rhabdomyosarcoma in the male may also originate elsewhere, such as in the urinary bladder or a bile duct. The tumour grows rapidly, is initially silent or causes only rather uncharacteristic clinical symptoms, e.g., hematuria, pain, urinary obstruction and infection. Therefore, even when detected relatively early, it has usually by then already involved both the bladder and the prostate, including the urethra (Fig. 3). It is sometimes impossible even histologically to determine the tumour origin with certainty. Metastases may affect the lymph nodes as well as the lungs, liver, spleen, peritoneum, and occasionally also the heart.

Radiologic diagnosis is based on the demonstration of a continuous soft tissue mass in the posterior part of the urethra and the base of the bladder. The urethra may be narrowed or dilated,

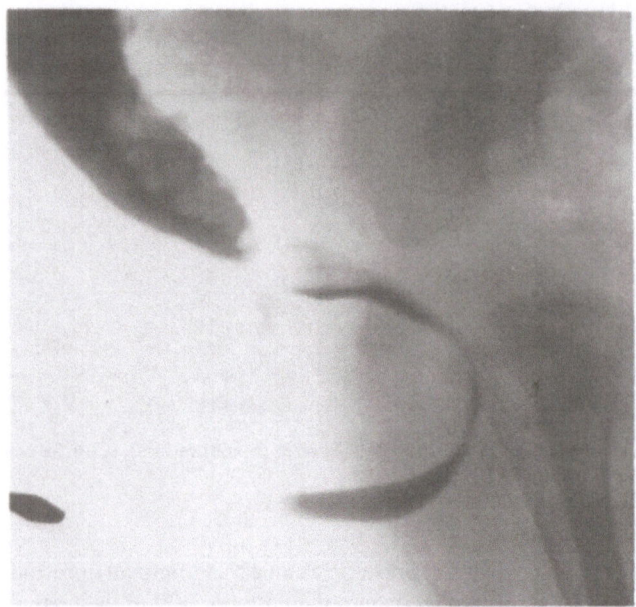

Fig. 3. Prostatic rhabdomyosarcoma. 6 months. UCG, lateral view. Slightly lobulated tumour intruding upon urethra and bladder from behind. (Courtesy of Dr. OLE EKLÖF)

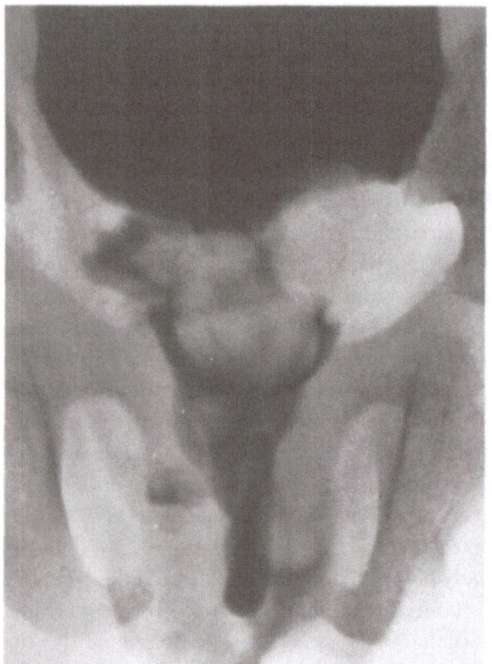

Fig. 4. Prostatic rhabdomyosarcoma. $2^1/_2$ years. UCG, a-p view. Lobulated tumour causing dilatation and ulceration of urethra and protruding into bladder. (Courtesy of Dr. OLE EKLÖF)

semble a bunch of grapes, an appearance which gave rise to its old name "sarcoma botryoides".

The radiologic findings in any type and stage of growth of the sarcoma may be mimicked by those in other abnormalities affecting both the urethra and the bladder. In the differential diagnosis one must sometimes consider possibilities such as an ectopic ureterocele or various unusual kinds of mucosal disease. These conditions will usually be recognized at complete radiologic exploration, but in doubtful cases biopsy is imperative.

4. The Prostatic Channels

4.1. Anomalous Channels

Two kinds of anomalous channels that may pierce the prostate from the outside and terminate in the urethra are diagnostically important in that they furnish valuable information on the major developmental anomaly in which they partake. These are the so-called fistula connecting the urethra with the bowel in certain cases of anorectal atresia, and the transprostatic ureter.

4.1.1. Bowel Fistula. This channel is probably the rudimentary terminal portion of the deficient rectum, but is conventionally referred to as a fistula.

sometimes also ulcerated (Figs. 3, 4). The surface of the tumour is, as a rule, lobulated early on (Fig. 3); when more advanced, the mass may re-

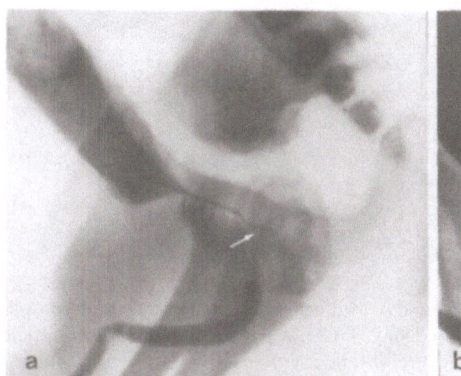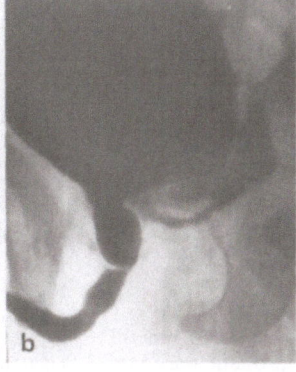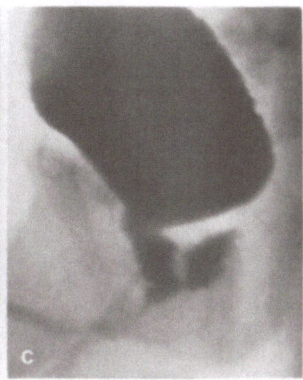

Fig. 5a-c. High anorectal atresia. a) 1 day. UCG (retrograde injection), lateral view. Angulation of urethra at site of narrow fistula *(arrow)*. No contrast medium in bowel. b) 8 months. UCG, oblique view. Contrast medium conveyed by fistula to bowel. c) 10 months. UCG, lateral view, 8 weeks after resection and closure of fistula. Postoperatively dilated fistula stump

It may reach the urethra at various levels in the male, but most often it enters the prostatic portion and thereby definitely classifies the malformation as high anorectal atresia. Without dwelling further on this point, it should be emphasized that classification is decisive for the choice of treatment and is essential also for the prognosis.

The urethral orifice of such a fistula is invariably in the posterior wall, and usually at the level of the seminal collicle, but in these cases the collicle may be less prominent than usual or even virtually absent. Traction exerted by the fistula tends instead to produce a fairly characteristic angulation of the posterior wall of the urethra, and sometimes of the anterior wall as well (Fig. 5). The fistula may be quite narrow and temporarily occluded by meconium and is then not easily filled with contrast medium (Fig. 5a). Under these circumstances the abnormal angulation of the urethra may be a valuable clue to the existence and site of the fistula [7]. In most cases, however, the fistula itself can be visualized at UCG or at least shown to convey contrast medium to the bowel (Fig. 5b).

It is, as a rule, also possible to demonstrate the fistula with contrast medium that has instead been introduced directly into the bowel after percutaneous puncture above the atretic portion [13]. This approach is becoming increasingly popular and has the advantage of providing optimal morphologic evaluation of the bowel. Successful puncture may be prohibited by the lack of gas in colon and rectum to guide the procedure, for example in cases where the intestinal tract is atretic also at some higher level.

Though the fistula may thus be initially explored without UCG, this method is required for proper postoperative examination. UCG after surgery is desirable because during reconstruction of the deficient bowel, which should include resection and closure of the fistula, a portion of the fistula at its urethral end may have been inadvertently or intentionally left behind as a residual pouch. This pouch tends to increase in size (Fig. 5c) and may cause considerable trouble requiring further surgery [1, 12].

4.1.2 Transprostatic Ureter. Any ectopic ureter, whether supernumerary or not, empties further caudally than an ordinary ureter. Its orifice may be in the bladder or urethra or outside the urinary pathways in both sexes, but in the male it cannot—for developmental reasons—open into the urethra at a level below the seminal collicle [5]. Hence, the terminal portion of any ureter emptying into the male urethra will reach its orifice by running either intramurally in the bladder neck and urethra or through the prostate.

In both cases the ureter is partly enclosed by the inner urethral sphincter and is thus compressed continuously except during voiding. This helps to explain the common occurrence of various complications apt to affect the entire ectopic urinary system. Such complications are beyond the scope of this review, but it should be remembered that

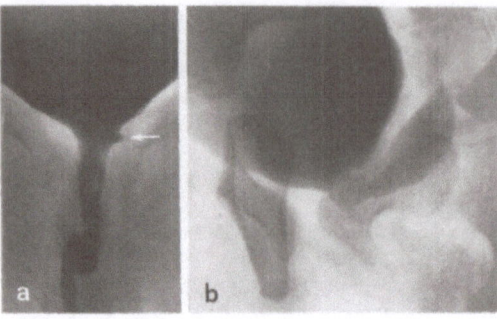

Fig. 6 a and b. Transprostatic ureter. a) 10 months. UCG, a-p view. Reflux to narrow prostatic portion of ectopic ureter *(arrow)*. UG at that time showed duplicated left renal pelvis with hydronephrotic upper compartment and dilated corresponding ureter but failed to demonstrate terminal ureteral portion, which was found at subsequent operation to be common to both left urinary systems. b) 14 months. UG, oblique view, 3 weeks after resection of dilated system. Ureterocele above orifice of ectopic ureter

they often include damage to the corresponding renal parenchyma and that UG may therefore fail to visualize the ectopic ureter. In some cases the ureter is demonstrated by reflux occurring during UCG, but even then it is not always possible to define every detail in the malformation preoperatively (Fig. 6).

4.2. Normally Existing Channels

The prostate normally contains the utricle, the ejaculatory ducts and a large number of glandular ducts.

4.2.1. The Utricle. Being a rudiment of the Müllerian ducts, the utricle corresponds to part of the vagina and uterus in the female. In the male fetus these ducts disappear almost completely, but their cloacal ends are converted into a pair of pockets in and behind the posterior wall of the urethra. The pockets normally fuse into one before birth, but they may remain separate, giving rise to a large utricle permanently divided into two compartments by a longitudinal septum (Fig. 7). This malformation is usually combined with hypospadias and may be considered a variety of intersexuality.

Also a nonseptate, large utricle may be a developmental anomaly. This, too, is found most fre-

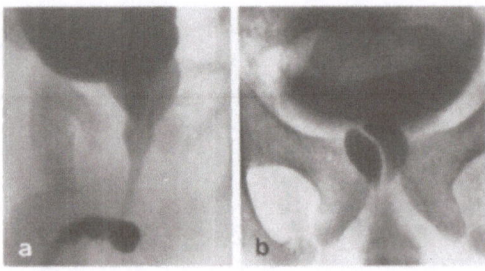

Fig. 7 a and b. Malformed utricle in boy with hypospadias. a) 1 day. UCG, a-p view. Large septate utricle behind urethra. b) 3 years. UCG, a-p view. Contrast medium retained in utricle after micturition

quently in hypospadias, but the anomaly occurs also as a component of the rare, so-called prune belly syndrome. However, a wide utricle may simply reflect dilatation caused, for example, by chronic urethral obstruction at any level distal to the seminal collicle (Fig. 8).

The normal utricle will usually not permit inflow of contrast medium at UCG, but when it does, it is seen to be only a minute pit at the center of the seminal collicle or a narrow channel extending a few millimeters toward the bladder in the midline behind the urethra. Any abnormally wide utricle, on the other hand, is likely to become visualized at UCG, and may retain contrast medium after cessation of micturition (Figs. 7 b, 8 b).

4.2.2. The Ejaculatory Ducts. These are also sometimes visible at UCG, most often in cases of urethral obstruction (Fig. 8). They run a caudal course not in, but close to, the midline behind the urethra to their orifices, which are situated in the collicle only slightly above or below that of the utricle. Therefore, if only one of the ducts is demonstrated it might be mistaken for a deep utricle. However, having entered one of these ducts, contrast medium usually proceeds into the corresponding *seminal vesicle*, which is easily recognized by its typically convoluted lumen (Fig. 8).

The vesicles are outside the prostate and extend craniolaterad close to the trigone of the bladder. They tend to retain contrast medium for a rather long time, whereas the ejaculatory ducts usually empty when, or even before, micturition is discontinued. A radiograph taken at UCG may therefore demonstrate the seminal vesicles without

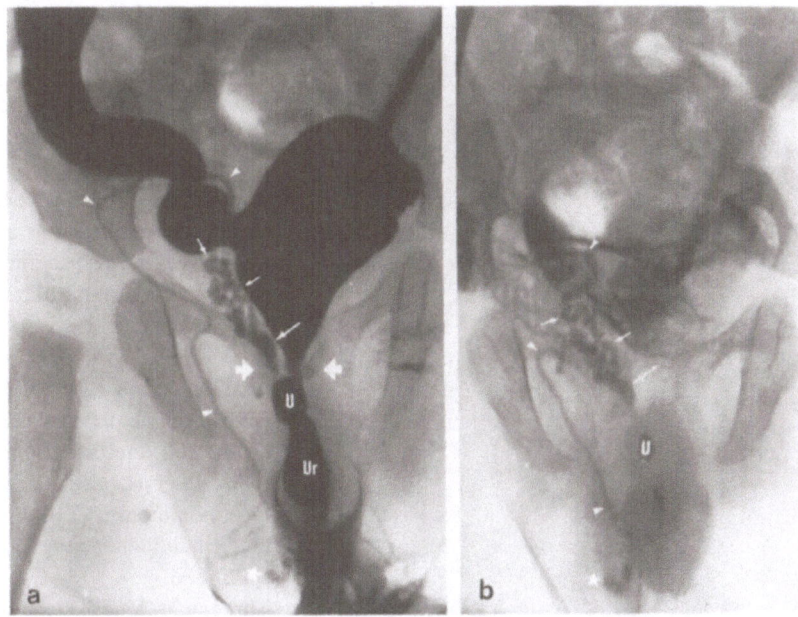

Fig. 8a and b. Congenital meatal stenosis of urethra. 10 months. UCG (suprapubic puncture), a-p views a) during, b) after, micturition. Wide urethra *(Ur)* and utricle *(U)*. Diverticula of bladder, reflux to dilated right ureter. Also note right ejaculatory duct *(long thin arrow)*, seminal vesicle *(short thin arrows)*, vas deferens *(arrowheads)*, epididymis *(asterisk)*, and bilateral prostatic ducts *(broad arrows)*

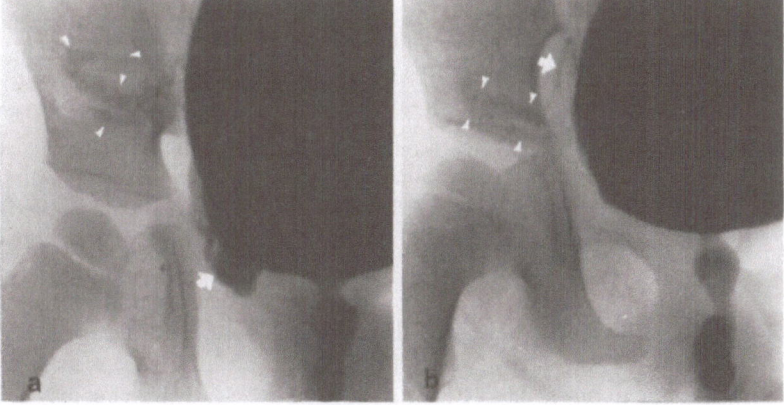

Fig. 9 a and b. Testis retention. 3 years. UCG, a-p views. Right epididymis at pelvic entrance *(arrowheads)*. Also note seminal vesicle *(arrow in a)* and vas deferens *(arrow in b)* but no visible ejaculatory duct. (Courtesy of Dr. ULF RUDHE)

showing the ejaculatory ducts (Fig. 9). Only rarely does the inflow of contrast medium continue into the *vas deferens*, but it may reach even the *epididymis* (Fig. 8). If this organ is thereby shown to be situated at the pelvic entrance, UCG has provided an unorthodox mode of diagnosing retention of the *testis* (Fig. 9).

4.2.3. The Glandular Ducts. The prostate develops from five separate epithelial buds in the primitive urethra and is accordingly divided into five lobes: an anterior lobe, a middle lobe, a posterior lobe, and two lateral lobes [6]. All of the many glandular ducts of the prostate proper are distributed within the lobes and may be referred to as

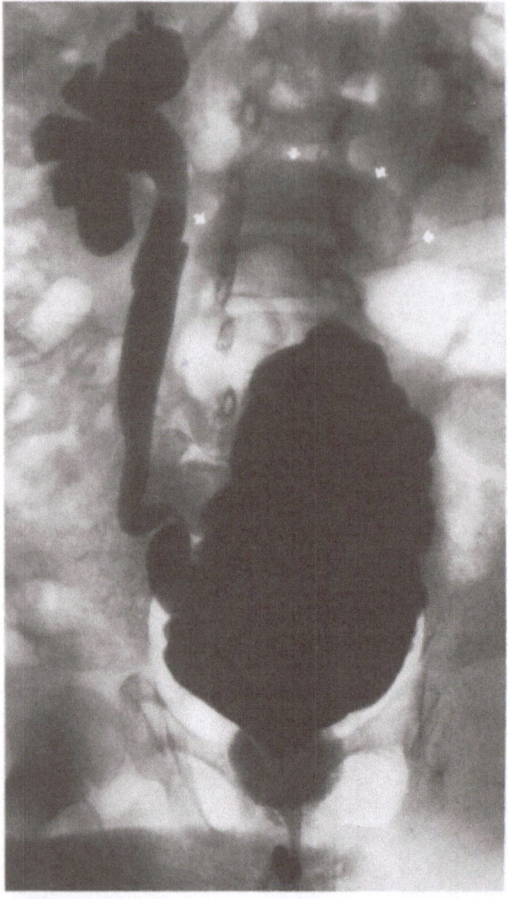

Fig. 10. Prostatic reflux in neurogenic disorder of bladder. 7 years. UCG, a-p view. Extensive reflux to virtually all glandular ducts of prostate. Note also spina bifida, myelomeningocele *(arrows)*, and dislocated left hip

lobar ducts. Other ducts, which are also numerous, are known as the *internal ducts* of the prostate but belong to tiny glands actually situated in the urethral mucosa. Similar periurethral glands exist also in parts of the urethra other than its prostatic portion. Furthermore, there are two specific groups of so-called *accessory prostatic ducts* outside the capsule of the prostate: one in the inner sphincter and the other in the trigonal mucosa.

The internal and accessory ducts seem never to have been visualized radiologically, but lobar ducts are frequently demonstrated by UCG at any age. In some cases contrast medium is seen to fill virtually all of these ducts even as far as the capsu-

lar border of the gland (Fig. 10), but more often only a few ducts are demonstrated (Figs. 8, 11, 12). They can often be radiologically assigned to specific lobes according to their site in various views [9]; the lateral lobes seem to be those most commonly affected.

The glandular ducts have minute flaps of tissue at their orifices, serving as a valve mechanism that normally prevents backflow from the urethra. The demonstration of the ducts at UCG thus indicates orificial insufficiency, or incompetence, of the ducts similar to that of the ureter in vesico-ureteral reflux. In view of this analogy it appears convenient to refer to retrograde filling of the glandular ducts of the prostate as prostatic reflux. Such reflux deserves particular interest because it is the most common of all radiologically demonstrable abnormalities affecting the prostate in infancy and childhood.

Three main kinds of conditions have been found to be separately or jointly responsible for prostatic reflux in children, viz., urethral obstruction below the level of the seminal collicle, neurogenic disorder of the urinary bladder, and urinary infection [10].

Urethral obstruction may overcome the normal valve mechanism at the ductal orifices by intermittently causing a brisk rise in pressure in the prostatic portion of the urethra during voiding. Prostatic reflux in children has been observed in obstruction due to a urethral valve (Fig. 11), a pedunculated collicular polyp, a urethral diverticulum, congenital stenosis of the urethral meatus (Fig. 8), or phimosis [10].

A neurogenic disorder of the bladder will also expose the orificial valve mechanism to abnormal pressure. The excess pressure is probably not particularly high but may be more or less continuous, because the inability to control the inner sphincter tends to be combined with deficient relaxation of the outer sphincter; this allows intravesical pressure, in severe cases, to be almost constantly transmitted to the prostate. The neurogenic disorders held responsible for prostatic reflux in children have in turn been caused by myelomeningocele (Fig. 10), neoplasm, or traumatic injury to the spinal cord [10, 11]. A maximal degree of prostatic reflux, like that shown in Figure 10, seems to have been observed exclusively in neurogenic disorders.

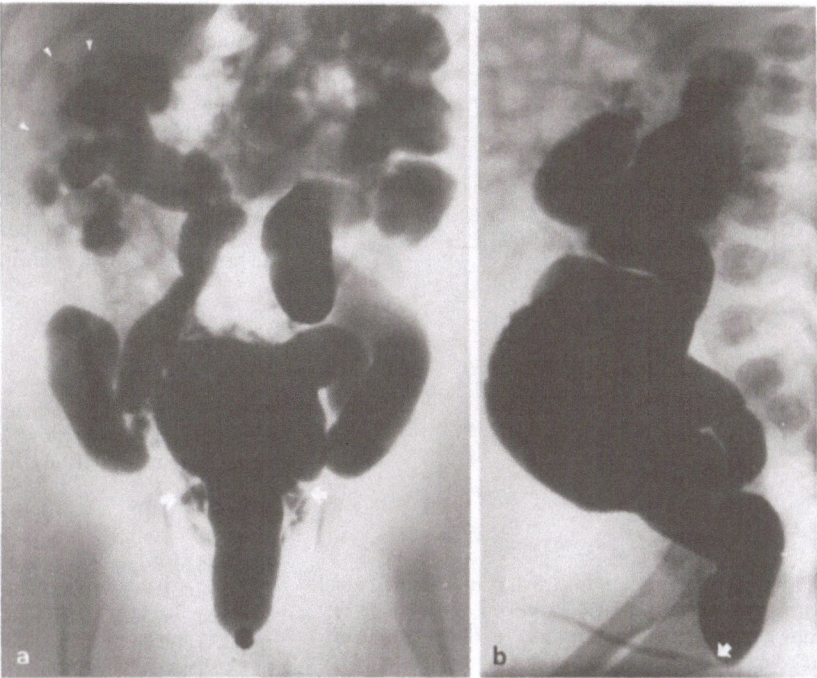

Fig. 11a and b. Prostatic reflux in urethral obstruction. 3 weeks. UCG, a) a-p, b) lateral, view. Reflux to dilated glandular ducts of prostate (*arrows in* a). Dilatation of entire urinary system above urethral valve (*arrow in* b), depressed to infraprostatic level during micturition. Bilateral vesicoureteral reflux including right renal tubular reflux *(arrowheads)*

Urinary infection may provoke prostatic reflux (Fig. 12) simply by causing inflammatory infiltration or edema of the urethral mucosa. This has a close analogy with the changes in cystitis which invite vesico-ureteral reflux.

Since, in fact, all three kinds of conditions favouring prostatic reflux also tend to provoke vesicoureteral reflux, it is not surprising that the latter abnormality and its various complications are common in children with prostatic reflux (Figs. 8, 10, 11). This might explain why prostatic reflux has received remarkably little attention. In the presence of much more spectacular and familiar findings, known to be clinically important, a few visible tiny ducts in the prostate may be thought rather irrelevant. Even in the absence of other radiologic findings, prostatic reflux will easily pass entirely unnoticed unless specifically sought for.

Urinary infection in any pediatric age group is far more frequent than either urethral obstruction or neurogenic disorders, and is a common complication of these conditions. One might therefore suspect that prostatic reflux in children is most often attributable to infection. This assumption was confirmed by the observations made in a series of 200 boys consecutively examined with UCG. Prostatic reflux was found in only 1 out of 69 cases without known infection (this boy had a neurogenic disorder), whereas the incidence in the group with urinary infection was more than 20% [11].

Prostatic reflux in urinary infection deserves attention not only because of its high incidence but especially because it indicates that the pathogenic microorganisms have access to the prostatic ducts. It has been shown in adults that bacteria lodging in these ducts often survive chemotherapy, because most such drugs do not pass in sufficient concentration through the tissues separating the ductal lumina from the prostatic blood vessels. The residual prostatitis after treatment for urinary infection in adults may produce no clinical symptoms, but it is considered a frequent cause of recurrence of manifest infection [8].

Infection of the prostatic ducts probably plays a similar role in children. The case history of the

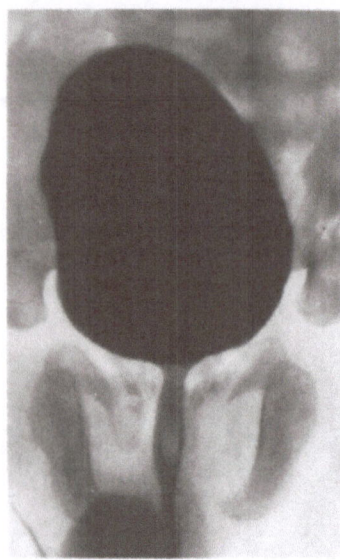

Fig. 12. Prostatic reflux in urinary infection (residual prostatitis). 6 weeks. UCG, a-p view. Reflux to a few tiny glandular ducts of prostate. Case history, see text. (From [11])

boy illustrated in Figure 12 lends support to this assumption. Prior to radiologic examination he had been treated for 5 weeks for urinary infection which had been preceded by neonatal urosepsis; urine samples obtained after each period of treatment had proved sterile. Because of the prostatic reflux detected at UCG urine was cultured again, but this time samples were taken both before and after massage of the prostate. Bacterial growth was found in the second fraction, but not in the first. Moreover, on all occasions the bacteria identified in this case proved to be of the same phage type of *Staphylococcus aureus*.

It is not known whether, or when, prostatic reflux might be expected to disappear after cure of urinary infection. In several cases repeated UCG has shown prostatic reflux to persist for years despite treatment, but most of these boys had urethral obstruction or a neurogenic disorder complicated by infection [10]. In children with prostatic reflux attributable to urinary infection alone, occasional reexamination after treatment has shown disappearance of the reflux in some cases but not in others [12]. A systematic radiologic and clinical follow-up of this category of cases is desirable, but this has not been undertaken as yet.

It is still uncertain whether prostatic reflux after treatment for urinary infection should be considered evidence of residual prostatitis or may have persisted despite healing of the infection. Whilst awaiting further research, the radiologic finding of prostatic reflux in patients undergoing such treatment should be considered an indication for culture of urine samples obtained after massage of the prostate before discontinuing therapy.

References

1. CURRARINO, G.: Diverticulum of prostatic urethra developing postoperatively from stump of congenital rectourethral fistula. Amer. J. Roentgenol. **106**, 211 (1969)
2. EDLING, N. P.: Urethrocystography in the male with special regard to micturition. Acta radiol. (Stockh.) Suppl. No. **51** (1945)
3. FIGDOR, P. P., WEISSENBACHER, G.: Prostatasteine bei einem vierjährigen Knaben. Zschr. Kinderchir. **7**, 293 (1969)
4. GULLMO, A., SUNDBERG, J.: A method for roentgen examination of the posterior urethra, prostatic ducts and utricle (utriculography). Acta radiol. (Stockh.) **48**, 241 (1957)
5. KJELLBERG, S. R., ERICSSON, N. O., RUDHE, U.: The Lower Urinary Tract in Childhood. Uppsala: Almqvist & Wiksell, 1957
6. LOWSLEY, O. S.: The development of the human prostate gland with reference to the development of other structures at the neck of the urinary bladder. Amer. J. Anat. **13**, 299 (1912)
7. RUDHE, U.: Congenital abnormalities of the large bowel. In: Encyclopedia of Medical Radiology, Vol. XI/2. Strnad, F. (ed.). Berlin, Heidelberg, New York: Springer-Verlag 1968
8. STAMEY, T. A., MEARES, E. M., WINNINGHAM, D. G.: Chronic bacterial prostatitis and the diffusion of drugs into prostatic fluid. J. Urol. (Baltimore) **103**, 187 (1970)
9. THEANDER, G.: Roentgen appearance of prostatic channels in infancy and childhood. Acta radiol. (Stockh.) (Diagnosis) **11**, 467 (1971)
10. THEANDER, G.: Abnormalities associated with orificial insufficiency of prostatic ducts in infants and children. Pediat. Radiol. **3**, 24 (1975)
11. THEANDER, G.: Relationship between urinary infection and insufficiency of prostatic ducts in infancy and childhood. Pediat. Radiol. **3**, 158 (1975)
12. THEANDER, G.: Unpublished observations
13. WAGNER, M. L., HARBERG, F. J., KUMAR, A. P. M., SINGLETON, E. B.: The evaluation of imperforate anus utilizing percutaneous injection of water-soluble iodide contrast material. Pediat. Radiol. **1**, 34 (1973)

Approaches to the Evaluation of the Hand in the Congenital Malformation Syndromes

A. K. Poznanski

1. Introduction

The hand has for many centuries been considered a mirror of disease. With Roentgen's discovery of X-rays, the hand was the first part of the human body to be studied radiologically. Within the first year of his discovery, many papers dealing with the radiologic diagnosis using the hand were published [9]. In 1896 SMITH [26] published a radiograph of a child with DOWN's syndrome; this was probably the first radiologic diagnosis of a congenital malformation syndrome.

Development of the hand occurs very early in fetal life. Even at the 7th to 9th week of gestation proportions of the hands are very similar to those of the adult [4] (Fig. 1). Many congenital anomalies of the hands such as clinodactyly [2] or carpal fusion [3] already occur in the developing fetus (Fig. 2) and may even be present at the mesenchymal stage of development.

When approaching the hand radiograph in evaluation of congenital malformation syndromes one should consider the hand from several points of view: 1. the overall form or shape of the hand skeleton; 2. evaluation of the size of the hand; 3. evaluation of osseous maturation.

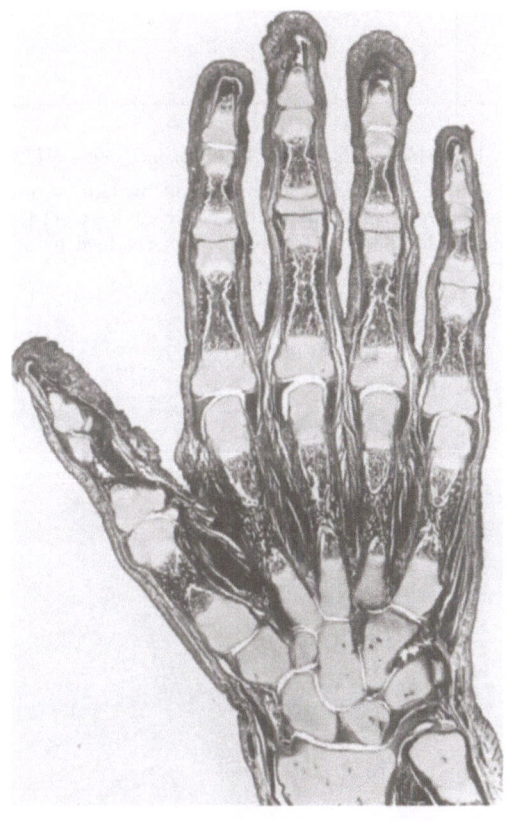

Fig. 1.a. Histologic section of hand of a 20-week black male fetus. When one considers cartilaginous as well as osseous portions of bone, proportions of hand bones appear remarkably similar to that of the adult. (Sections courtesy of Dr. Al Burdi, Department of Anatomy, University of Michigan)

2. Alterations in Configuration of the Hand Bones

Many of the observed alterations in the configuration of the hand bones are not pathognomonic; however, they are usually limited to only a few syndromes, and may thus aid in diagnosis. Lists of syndromes with these various anomalies have been published [13, 22, 25]. These lists may be diagnostically useful in a specific case as they significantly narrow down the diagnostic possibilities. Thus, if a certain anomaly is present one can decide that the patient falls into a certain group of disorders. On examining the list many diagnoses

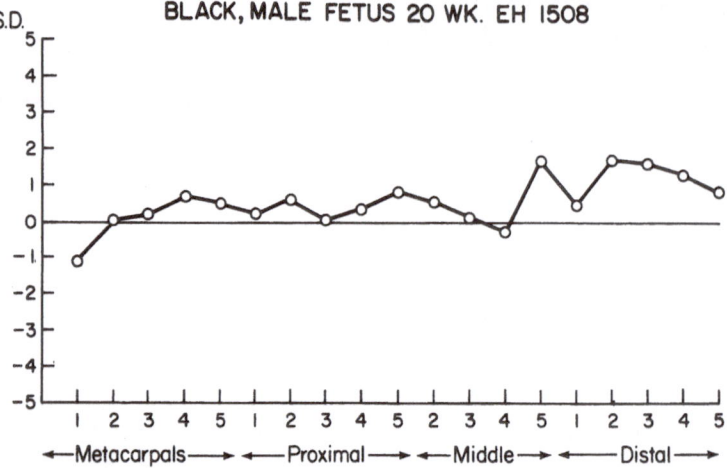

BLACK, MALE FETUS 20 WK. EH 1508

Fig. 1. b. Pattern profile analysis of this fetus shows considerable similarity to that of the adult except for distal phalanges. Pattern profile was obtained by as-signing metacarpal 2 the mean adult size and other bones were then adjusted appropriately

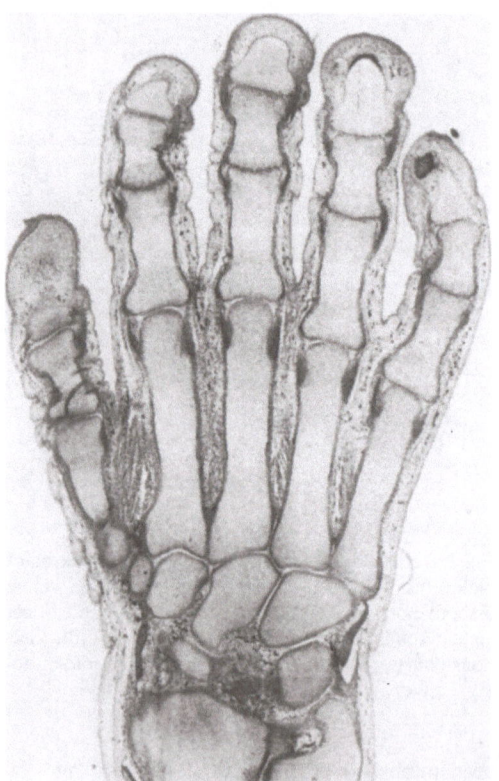

Fig. 2. Longitudinal section of a 50 mm male fetus. Hands are still at the cartilaginous phase except for a very minimal ossification of distal portion of fourth distal phalangeal tuft. Note that the cartilaginous model of middle phalanx of fifth finger shows evidence of clinodactyly, with the radial side being smaller than the ulnar. (Histologic sections courtesy of Dr. AL BUR-DI, Department of Anatomy, University of Michigan)

can be eliminated either clinically or by the presence of other associated abnormalities of the hand or other portions of the skeleton. Figure 3 illustrates such an example. Here we see the association of polydactyly and cone-shaped epiphyses. Although there are many disorders that can occur with either polydactyly or cone-shaped epiphyses [13], when one compares the two lists, the main condition that remains is chondroectodermal dysplasia, of which this is an example. Similarly, the importance of making the association between the hand findings and the clinical findings is illustrated in Figure 4. Here we see polydactyly which alone is fairly nonspecific and may be commonly present as an isolated finding. However, in this case we know that the child had a midline facial cleft. When one compares the list of disorders with midline facial clefts and the list with polydactyly, the number of syndromes considered is significantly decreased and the only condition that really fits is trisomy 13, which is indeed the diagnosis of this patient.

There are a number of alterations in configuration of the hand that may be diagnostically useful:

Shape of Bones. Evaluation of unusual shapes of bones requires subjective evaluation and knowledge of the various patterns that exist. A number of patterns appear fairly typical, for example in metatropic dwarfism (Fig. 5), the drumstick appearance of the bones is very suggestive of this disorder. Similarly, pointing of the ends of the

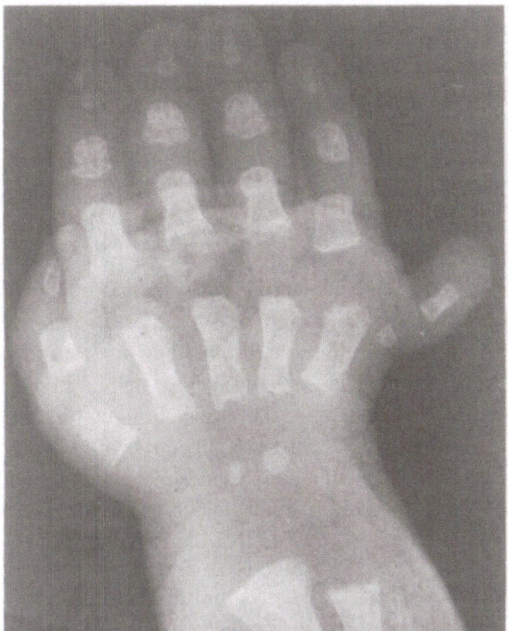

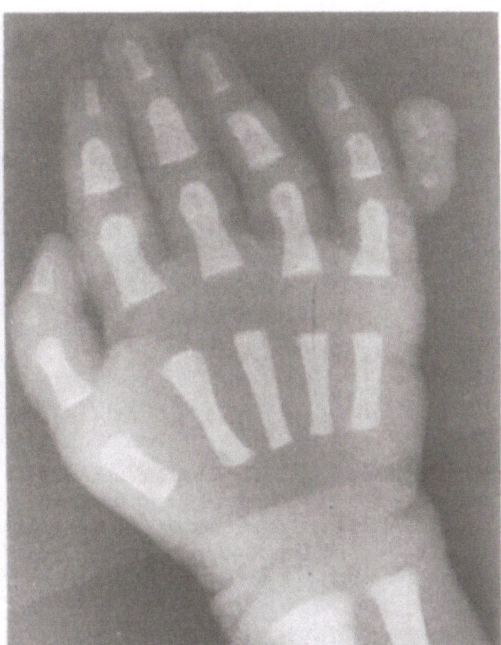

Fig. 3. Chondroectodermal dysplasia. There is poly-dactyly of the post-axial type. Note also characteristic appearance of distal phalanges, which appear very thin, and cone like indentations at bases of proximal phalanges. The combination of these findings is diag-nostic of chondroectodermal dysplasia

Fig. 4. Polydactyly in trisomy 13. This type of postaxial polydactyly can often be seen as a normal variant. However, the presence of a large mid-line facial cleft noted in this infant, together with polydactyly, sug-gests diagnosis of trisomy 13. Note also extra ossicle in thumb. Triphalangeal thumb has sometimes been seen in trisomy 13, but is not a common finding

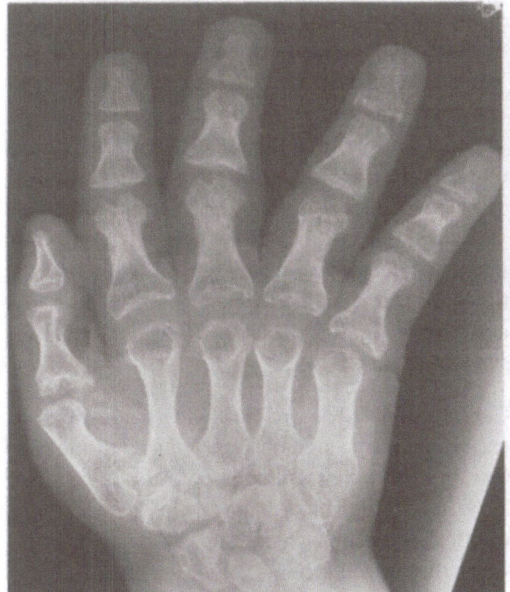

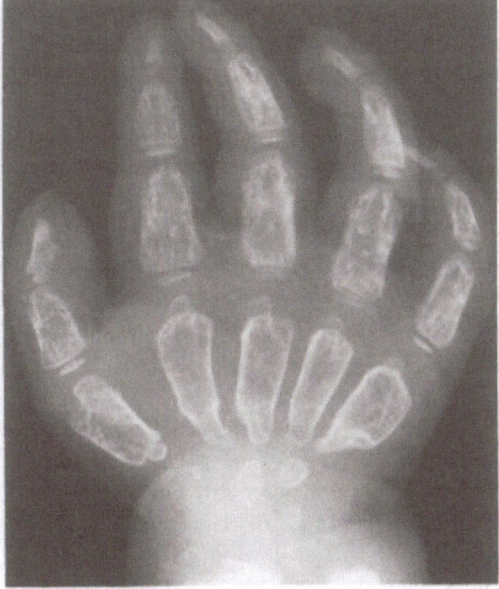

Fig. 5. Metatropic dwarfism. Middle phalanges and proximal phalanges have narrow waists and a some-what drumstick appearance. This is very suggestive of metatropic dwarfism

Fig. 6. I-cell disease. Sharp, pointed proximal metacar-pals and abnormalities in bone modelling are charac-teristic of the mucopolysaccharidosis-mucolipodosis group

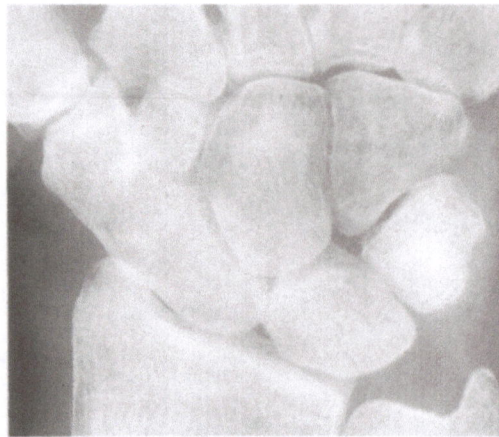

Fig. 7. Trapezium-scaphoid fusion in a patient with the hand-foot-genital syndrome. This type of carpal fusion, which goes across rows, indicates that patient has some congenital malformation syndrome. This type of fusion does not occur in the normal population

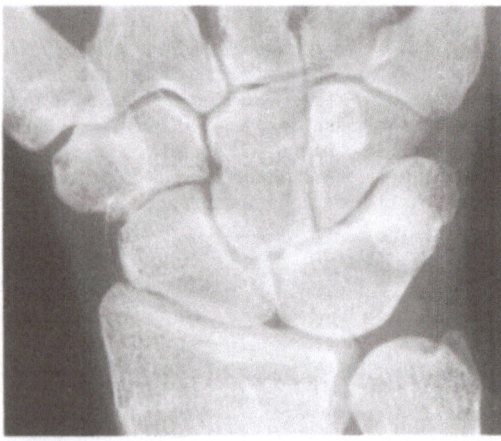

Fig. 8. Triquetrum-lunate fusion. This type of fusion may occur in normal individuals, particularly among blacks. It can also occur in congenital abnormalities

bones may be seen in a large group of mucopolysaccharidoses and mucolipidosis such as in this child with I-cell disease illustrated in Figure 6. This appearance of dysostosis multiplex is nonspecific for the type of mucopolysaccharide disturbance involved, however, by knowing the age of the patient and the associated clinical findings one can again narrow down the diagnostic possibilities.

Bone Modelling. There are a number of disorders which are associated with disturbances of bone

modelling. The above described I-cell disease is such an example and this finding may be seen in other mucopolysaccharide disturbances as well. Other disorders may cause either over modelling or under modelling of bone.

Bone Density. Very opaque or very lucent bones may be present in some congenital malformation syndromes. For example, increased bone density may be seen in osteopetrosis, pyknodysostosis, sclerosteosis, and endosteal hyperostosis, as well as in several other conditions. The association of other findings in the hand may be helpful in diagnosis. For example, the association of tuft erosions with bone sclerosis is suggestive of pyknodysostosis [13] while the presence of syndactyly and deviation of the second digit in association with bone sclerosis is suggestive of sclerosteosis [13].

Polydactyly. Many congenital malformation syndromes may be associated with polydactyly. When evaluating polydactyly it is important to determine whether it is on the preaxial or on the postaxial side of the hand since different syndromes are associated with each of these locations [13]. Also, certain syndromes may be associated with polydactyly involving the central portion of the hand. This is a much rarer association.

Syndactyly. Cutaneous syndactyly is a clinical diagnosis, but if severe it may be seen radiographically. Osseous syndactyly, on the other hand, is an important radiologic finding. Some forms of osseous syndactyly are associated with congenital syndromes [13]. For example, the acrocephalosyndactyly syndromes may have characteristic patterns of osseous syndactyly. There are also other disorders with milder forms of syndactyly and both sporadic and familial forms of isolated syndactyly may be seen.

Carpal Fusions. The presence of carpal fusion is a useful diagnostic sign of some congenital malformation syndromes. The type of fusion is particularly important since it may help to determine whether one is dealing with a syndrome. The fusions that involve bones of different rows, i.e., proximal to distal such as the trapezium-scaphoid fusion (Fig. 7) or the capitate-lunate fusion are almost invariably associated with some sort of congenital malformation syndrome [13, 19]. On the other hand, fusions involving bones of the same row may be associated with syndromes or may occur as isolated variants that are much less useful diagnostically [13]. For example, triquetrum-lunate fusion (Fig. 8) is a relatively common isolated fusion, particularly among black people; it was seen in 1.6% of such Americans [6]. In evaluation of carpal fusion, again the presence of other anomalies of the hand may be diagnostically useful. In Figure 9, there is a combination of fusion of the trapezium and scaphoid and a broad distal phalanx of the thumb with a cone epiphysis as well as a transverse capitate. This combination is diagnostic of the oto-palato-digital syndrome [20].

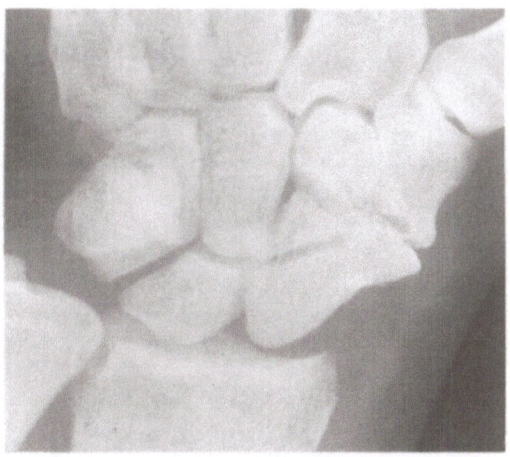

Fig. 10. Os centrale in patient with the Holt-Oram syndrome. Small ossicle between scaphoid and capitate is normally not present in man. The presence of this ossicle is suggestive of a number of syndromes of which the Holt-Oram is one of the most important. Note also the narrowing between trapezium-scaphoid which, just as fusion, is a sign of association with a congenital malformation syndrome

Accessory Carpals. Although most accessory carpal bones are of little diagnostic value, two are particularly important. These are the os centrale and os triangulare. The os centrale is particularly important as it is associated with a limited number of congenital malformation syndromes including the Holt-Oram syndrome [13, 14] (Fig. 10) and the hand-foot-genital syndrome. Presence of this ossicle is thus a very important and useful sign of congenital malformation syndromes.

Carpal Angle. The relative position of the carpals may have some diagnostic value. The carpal angle was defined as the angle formed by the intersection of a line tangent to the proximal edge of the lunate and scaphoid and a line tangent to the proximal edge of the lunate and triquetrum. Although the angle was first described in Turner syndrome [10], we have found that this is not a very good sign of this disease [18]. There are however a number of syndromes with increased carpal angle in which this sign may be useful in diagnosis particularly some of the epiphyseal dysplasias and arthrogryposis [18]. When measuring the carpal angle it is important that the hand be in neutral

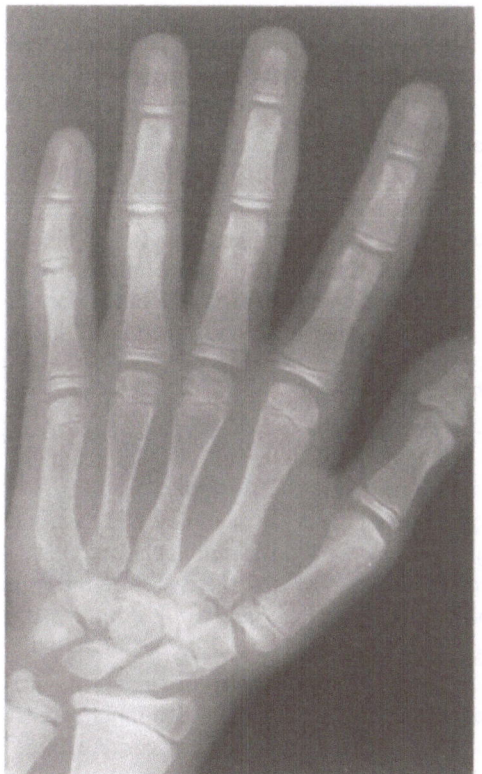

Fig. 9. Hand in the oto-palato-digital syndrome. Here we see association of trapezium-scaphoid fusion with a very broad distal phalanx of the thumb with an unusual cone epiphysis. This combination is very suggestive of the oto-plato-digital syndrome. Other findings of this condition include an abnormal base of the second metacarpal and a somewhat transverse capitate

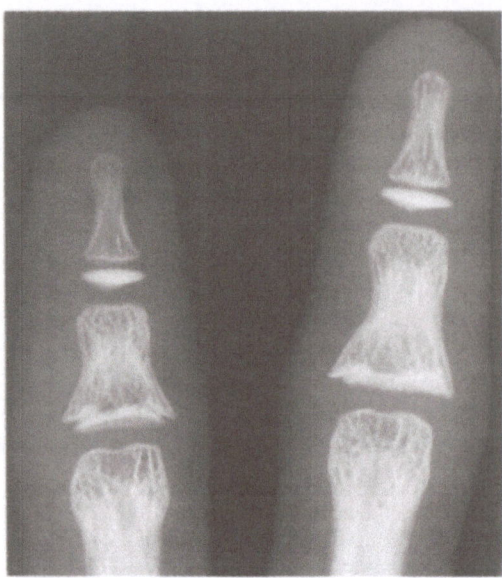

Fig. 11. Cone epiphyses and ivory epiphyses in the trichorhinophalangeal syndrome. The ivory epiphyses are sclerotic dense epiphyses seen here in distal phalanges. The type of cone epiphyses seen here in middle phalanges is characterized by fusion to the middle of the metaphyses and is associated with splaying of the metaphysis. The type of cone is fairly typical of the trichorhinophalangeal syndrome

position as ulnar or radial deviation can alter this angle [18].

Symphalangism. This is a disorder in which there is fusion of a phalanx to another phalanx within the same digit. Although symphalangism may occur as an isolated familial variant associated with carpal and tarsal fusion, it may also be seen in a number of congenital malformation syndromes, particularly some of the acrocephalosyndactyly disorders [12].

Triphalangeal Thumb. This is an extremely rare normal variant which has been associated with a number of syndromes [13], the most important of which is the Holt-Oram [14]. Triphalangeal thumbs may be seen in thalidomide embryopathy and also in the Blackfan-Diamond anemia. In the triphalangeal thumb the thumb has a third phalanx and frequently has a fingerlike appearance.

Curvature of the Fingers. Clinodactyly is the most common type of curved finger. The term clinodac-

tyly indicates a deviation of the finger in the medial lateral plane, usually it refers to the radial deviation of the fifth finger. This entity is often associated with a short middle phalanx and is extremely common in the normal population with an incidence of 1–25% depending on the population studied [13]. It is also seen in a large number of congenital malformation syndromes [13]. It is thus of little value diagnostically unless it is associated with other radiographic or clinical findings. However, in some cases the association may be of value such as, for example, in Silver syndrome where presence of clinodactyly and asymmetry in maturation and size of the two hands may very well suggest this syndrome.

Epiphyseal Abnormalities. A number of epiphyseal abnormalities have diagnostic value. These include cone epiphyses, ivory epiphyses, multiple epiphyseal ossification centers and pseudoepiphyses. Although many of these may be present as normal variants some are syndrome associated.

Cone epiphyses are defined as epiphyses which have projections towards the center of the metaphysis. A great variety of these cone epiphyses may be seen. Giedion has classified cone epiphyses into 38 types [6, 8]. Some of these types are seen as normal variants, while others are due to trauma or other unknown or acquired factors. A few types of cone epiphyses are typical of specific congenital malformation syndromes. For example, type 24 of the distal phalanges and types 19 and 20 of the middle phalanges are pathognomonic of cleidocranial dysostosis. Type 38 is quite suggestive of chondroectodermal dysplasia while type 12 is seen in the trichorhinophalangeal syndrome (Fig. 11). Sometimes even before the cone epiphyses are apparent indentations in the metaphyses are quite suggestive of a cone (Fig. 4).

Ivory epiphyses are very sclerotic epiphyses which may be seen in 0.35% of the U.S. normal population [11] and are particularly associated with delayed skeletal maturation. They may also be seen in association with several syndromes, particularly the Cockayne and the trichorhinophalangeal (Fig. 11). They may also be seen in some of the epiphyseal dysplasias.

Pseudoepiphyses may be seen as normal variants particularly when they involve the proximal portions of the metacarpals. When present in large numbers however, they are very suggestive of a syndrome. For example, in Wolfe syndrome [13], pseudoepiphyses usually involve all of the bones of the hand.

Absence Deformities of the Hand. The absence defects may be related to syndromes or may be familial without other abnormalities, or may be sporadic. Differentiation between the various types cannot always be made radiologically. The defects may be terminal, appearing as an amputation, or may involve one portion of the hand, for example the radial or the ulnar. Generally speaking, the radial defects such as absences of the thumb, are more commonly syndrome associated or concomitants of some additional congenital anomalies such as those of the heart, head, neck: defects of the ulnar side of the hand are more commonly sporadic [13]. However, both types of defect may be seen as isolated findings.

3. Evaluation of the Size of the Hand Bones

Determination of shortening or lengthening of the bones of the hand is very useful in diagnosis of congenital malformation syndromes, and has

been used both clinically and radiologically for some time. In the hand it is convenient to consider each segment separately. For example, there are a number of syndromes where the distal phalanges are affected or else the middle phalanges or the metacarpals. Other disorders are associated with shortening on either the radial or ulnar side of the hand. As in the absence defects, the radial shortenings are more frequently syndrome associated than the ulnar. When alterations in length of the hand bones are extreme, only simple observation of the radiograph is needed to determine whether a bone is indeed shortened (Fig. 12), and reference to appropriate tables of what disorders are associated with which type of shortening will often yield the diagnosis. Frequently, however, the shortening is more subtle, and other methods of evaluation must be used. These methods include shortcuts such as the metacarpal sign, or more sophisticated methods such as the use of ratios and pattern profiles.

3.1. The Metacarpal Sign

This is a simple sign that was described to evaluate shortening of the fourth metacarpal. It was described by ARCHIBALD [1] and is produced by drawing a line tangential to the heads of the fifth

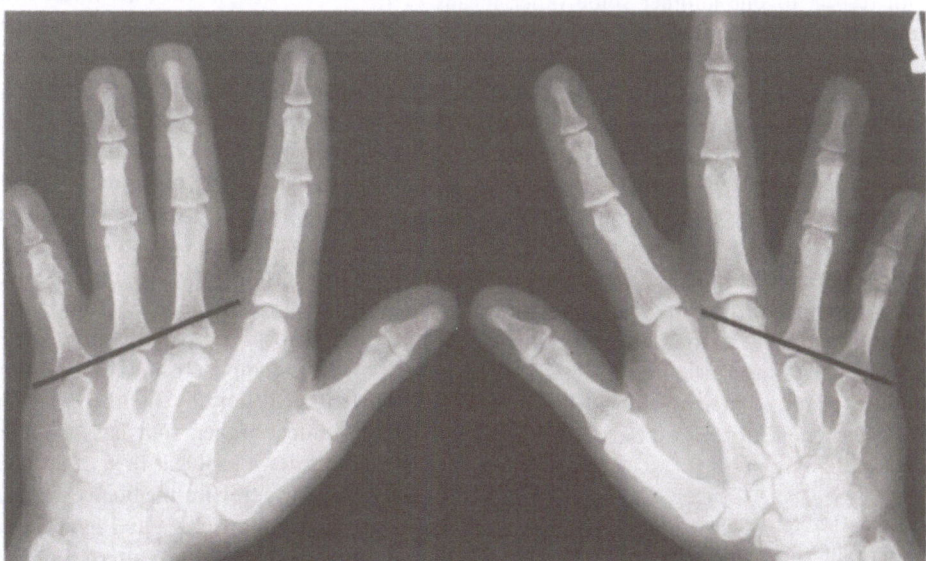

Fig. 12. Metacarpal sign in an XO Turner. On the left, metacarpal sign is negative because third metacarpal is also short. On the right it is positive

and forth metacarpals (Fig. 12). Normally, this line does not intersect the third. When the fourth metacarpal is short, this line will usually intersect the third metacarpal and will then be positive. The sign, however, is not very reliable since it is positive in almost 10% of the normal population [24] and is also very dependent upon the relative shortening of the third and fifth metacarpals. For example, in Figure 12 the metacarpal sign is negative on the left hand in spite of marked shortening of the fourth. This is due to the fact that the third is also shortened. On the right the metacarpal sign is positive. Similarly, if the fifth metacarpal was shortened as much or more than the fourth there may be a negative metacarpal sign as well. Thus false negative metacarpal signs may be seen in spite of obvious shortening of the fourth.

3.2. Bone Length Measurements

Normal standards for length of the hand bones have been derived by Garn for a white population [5]. However, the measurements per se will not determine when a bone is relatively short. The patient himself may be relatively small or may have relatively small but symmetrically shortened hands. To determine the relative size of the bones with respect to one another some other means have to be used. The methods we have used include ratios, or pattern profiles.

Ratios. An elegant way to determine the relative length of one bone as compared to another is to use bone length ratios. The values for the ratios of the length of each bone to every other bone and the standard deviation of variation for this ratio have been published [13]. Thus, any two bones can be compared, and one can determine how deviant the ratios are from the mean. However, it is difficult and time consuming to obtain the large number of ratios that are possible when one compares each bone to every other bone, so other methods have been sought.

Pattern Profile Analysis. Since it is the relative amount of shortening that needs to be determined, one could compare one bone to another in terms of how deviant each is from the norm. Thus,

one could determine by how many standard deviations each of the hand bones deviates from the mean. This is the "Z-score." Comparison of Z-score of one bone to the Z-score of another can be done by simply comparing the figures, although it is difficult to visualize the relative size of each of the hand bones by this method. The pattern profile approach [17] in essence is a graphic display of this relative shortening and lengthening of each of the hand bones.

In this method, the length of each of the hand bones is measured with a direct reading caliper and compared to the norms for age and sex [5]. The number of standard deviations that each of the bones deviates from the norm for the specific age and sex is then determined (Z-score). The Z-score is then plotted in the ordinate against the location in the hand on the abscissa (Fig. 13). Thus, one obtains a visual display of the relative size of each bone to every other bone [17]. With this technique one can compare males against females and patients of different ages with one another (Fig. 13). Also mean patterns can be obtained for specific syndromes so that an individual can be compared to the mean for a certain disorder (Fig. 13). We have now developed means for approximately 100 congenital malformation syndromes. In some of these, the number of cases was quite large and an accurate mean could be obtained. Certainly not all syndromes have a specific or pathognomonic pattern of hand abnormality, but often only a few syndromes will have a similar mean, so that the pattern will be suggestive of a small group of syndromes which can then be separated by clinical or other means. For example, when the computer was used to determine the patterns that were most similar to the hand-foot-genital syndromes, it was found that myositis ossificans progressiva and the campomelique syndromes had similar patterns (Fig. 14). These syndromes are completely different and can easily be differentiated clinically. In other syndromes a very large number of them may have a similar pattern and the pattern profile is then of little value. This is particularly true for the bone dysplasias, particularly in achondroplasia and hypochondroplasia. In other syndromes, the pattern is essentially normal and it therefore has no diagnostic value, as in the Schmidt type of metaphyseal dysostosis.

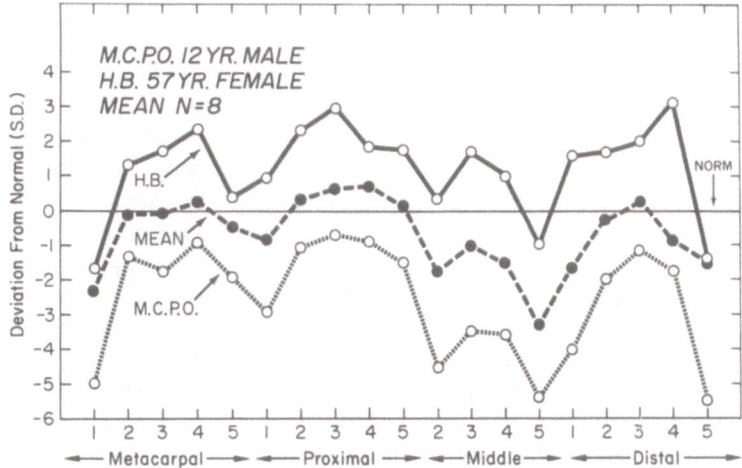

Fig. 13. Pattern profiles, hand-foot-genital syndrome. Here we see a plot of relative alterations in hand length of an adult female, H.B., a 12-year-old boy, M.C.P.O., and the mean for the syndrome. This graph plots number of standard deviations from normal length of each of the hand bones according to location in the hand. Note remarkable similarity of patterns between these individuals and their similarity to the mean. Height of pattern in relationship to zero line simply indicates whether the hand is smaller or larger than the mean. Thus, adult female had a relatively large hand for her age while 12-year-old boy had a relatively small hand. However, the ups and downs of the pattern are remarkably alike. On looking at the original radiographs, short first metacarpals and middle phalanges of the fingers could be visualized, but the other shortenings could not be identified by simple inspection

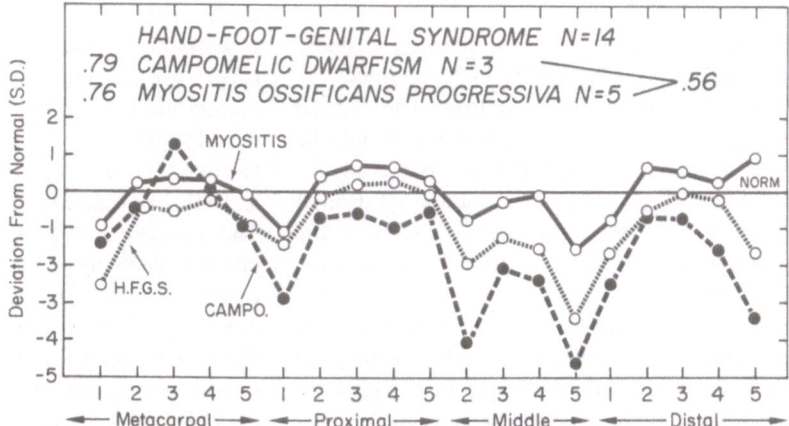

Fig. 14. Comparisons of patterns in several different syndromes. There is considerable similarity between the hand-foot-genital syndrome and campomelic dwarfism and myositis ossificans progressiva. However, these syndromes can be simply differentiated by other clinical manifestations

3.3. Bone Quality

The amount of bone in the second metacarpal may be altered in the congenital malformation syndrome. Certainly children with chronic disease or many of the congenital malformation syndromes have a decrease in the amount of bone. To determine the amount of bone in the second metacarpal both its outside diameter, T, and its inside diameter, M, are measured at its mid-portion. With these measurements one can obtain the cortical thickness, $C = T - M$ and the percent cortical area, $PCA = T^2 - M^2/T^2$. By the use of these measurements and comparison to the norms [7] one can determine disorders in which there is more endosteal or subperiosteal resorption or apposition. It appears that different congenital malformations may have different ways in which they affect these factors [7].

3.4. Slenderness Ratios

PARISH [12], and SINCLAIR et al. [23] describe the use of slenderness ratio in the diagnosis of conditions where relative thinning of the bone has occurred, such as in Marfan syndrome. To determine this, the length of a bone is divided by its width. In our experience this has not been a very useful measurement in the diagnosis of Marfan syndrome, since a number of patients with classic Marfan syndrome have a normal ratio.

4. Determination of Skeletal Maturation

Skeletal maturation has little meaning in disorders with gross abnormality of bone, since it is very difficult to match or compare it to normal standards, and standards of maturation for the bone dysplasias or syndromes are not available. However, in congenital malformation syndromes where architecture is not greatly disturbed, the determination of skeletal maturation can be diagnostically useful.

In most congenital malformation syndromes, skeletal maturation is retarded, so that retardation itself is not much value in diagnosis. The presence of advanced maturation, particularly in the newborn, is more useful since the list of conditions with advancement in this age group is very small [16] and diagnosis is limited to such conditions as the Marshall syndrome, the Weaver syndrome, and infantile hyperthyroidism. In older children, advancement of maturation in the presence of mental retardation may be useful as it is very uncommon, and its presence is a possible sign of cerebral giantism [15, 21]. In determining skeletal maturation one should determine not only whether it is advanced or retarded but also whether there is evidence of disharmonic maturation, and if so, of which type [16].

Frequently, in the congenital malformation syndrome, the maturation does not fit with the usual pattern of ossification as seen in the standard atlases. This lack of fit to the more common pattern has been termed "disharmonic maturation" [15]. Disharmony may be considered in various ways, including alteration in sequence of ossification, comparison between carpals and phalanges, or relative advancement or retardation of specific centers [16]. Sequence alterations occur much more commonly in the congenital malformation syndromes than in normal children. For example, 718 sequences were seen in congenital malformation syndromes, while in the much larger group of normal children 622 different sequences were observed. Ninty-seven sequences were seen only in the congenital malformation syndrome group [16].

Comparison between the phalanges and carpals is a useful way to look at skeletal maturation. Some differences between the two areas exist in a normal population; however, when the differences are gross they may have diagnostic value. Generally speaking, when skeletal age is advanced the carpals are ahead of the phalanges [16, 27]. When maturation is retarded they appear behind. This would suggest that the carpals are more sensitive to alterations in maturation. A few exceptions exist to this rule, and may be diagnostically useful. The main one is cerebral giantism where, in spite of advanced maturation, the phalanges are significantly and consistently ahead of the carpals [15, 21].

Delay of certain ossification centers can occur in a number of syndromes; for example, hypoplasia of the radial carpals such as the trapezium and trapezoid is seen in syndromes associated with radial hypoplasia. Delay of the scaphoid may be seen in cerebral giantism, a late lunate has been described in homocystinuria, and other relative delays have also been described [13, 16]. Advancement of local centers is less common. Asymmetry in maturation is another form of disharmony seen in conditions with asymmetry in size such as hemihypertrophy in Silver syndrome. Lists of the syndromes with various types of disharmony have been published [16].

5. Summary

The hand has always been considered a mirror of disease, and similarly the hand radiograph is also frequently the mirror of disease, particularly in the congenital malformation syndromes. Of all of the portions of the skeleton, the hand probably yields the most diagnostic information in systemic disease. This is partially because of our extensive knowledge of the normal variability in the hand, and the fact that it contains both round and long bones.

When evaluating the hand we have to look not only at the various anomalies but also at certain normal variants, since these may be diagnostically useful. By considering the patterns of both anomalies and variants, the diagnosis of a specific congenital malformation syndrome or at least a group of congenital malformation syndromes can often be made. When the hand findings are combined with patterns of anomalies in the remainder of the skeleton, or with additional clinical findings, correct diagnosis becomes more likely. Certainly the hand should not be considered alone without correlation to these other areas.

Measurements of the hand bones are an additional approach which has proved very useful in detecting subtle alterations in bone lengths or bone mass. The length measurements are particularly useful when used in combination with the pattern profile method.

References

1. ARCHIBALD, R. M., FINBY, N., DE VITO, F.: Endocrine significance of short metacarpals. J. Clin. Endocrinol. Metabol. 19, 1312—1322 (1959)

2. GARN, S. M., BABLER, W. J., BURDI, A. R.: Prenatal origins of brachymesophalangia-5. Am. J. Phys. Anthrop. 44 413—416 (1976)

3. GARN, S. M., BURDI, A. R., BABLER, W. J.: Prenatal origins of carpal fusions. Am. J. Phys. Anthrop. 45, 203—207 (1976)

4. GARN, S. M., BURDI, A. R., BABLER, W. J., STINSON, S.: Early prenatal attainment of adult metacarpal-phalangeal rankings and proportions. Am. J. Phys. Anthrop. 43, 327—332 (1975)

5. GARN, S. M., FRISANCHO, A. R., POZNANSKI, A. K., SCHWEITZER, J., MCCANN, M. B.: Analysis of triquetral-lunate fusion. Am. J. Phys. Anthrop. 34, 431—434 (1971)

6. GARN, S. M., HERTZOG, K. P., POZNANSKI, A. K., NAGY, J. M.: Metacarpo-phalangeal length in the evaluation of skeletal malformation. Radiology 105, 375—381 (1972)

7. GARN, S. M., POZNANSKI, A. K., NAGY, J. M.: Bone measurement in the differential diagnosis of osteopenia and osteoporosis. Radiology 100, 509—518 (1971)

8. GIEDION, A.: Zapfenepiphysen. Naturgeschichte und diagnostische Bedeutung einer Störung des enchondralen Wachstums. In: GLAUNER, R., RÜTTIMANN, A., THURN, P., VOGLER, E. (eds.): Ergebnisse der Medizinischen Radiologie. Stuttgart: Georg Thieme Verlag 1968

9. GRIGG, E. R. N.: In: BRUWER, A. J. (ed.): Classic Descriptions in Roentgenology. Vol. I, pp. 47—70, Springfield, Ill.: Charles C. THOMAS 1964

10. KOSOWICZ, J.: Roentgen appearance of hand and wrist in gonadal dysgenesis. Am. J. Roentgenol. 93, 354—361 (1965)

11. KUHNS, L. R., POZNANSKI, A. K., HARPER, H. A. S., GARN, S. M.: Ivory epiphyses of the hands. Radiology 109, 643—648 (1973)

12. PARISH, J. G.: Skeletal hand charts in inherited connective tissue disease. J. Med. Genet. 4, 227—238 (1967)

13. POZNANSKI, A. K.: The Hand in Radiologic Diagnosis. Philadelphia: W. B. SAUNDERS 1974

14. POZNANSKI, A. K., GALL, J. C., JR., STERN, A. M.: Skeletal manifestations of the Holt-Oram syndrome. Radiology 94 45—53 (1970)

15. POZNANSKI, A. K., GARN, S. M., KUHNS, L. R., SANDUSKY, S. T.: Dysharmonic maturation of the hand in the congential malformation syndromes. Am. J. Phys. Anthrop. 35, 417—432 (1971)

16. POZNANSKI, A. K., GARN, S. M., KUHNS, L. R., SHAW, H. A.: Disharmonic skeletal maturation in the congenital malformation syndromes. Birth Defects: Original Article Series (in press)

17. POZNANSKI, A. K., GARN, S. M., NAGY, J. M., GALL, J. C. JR.: Metacarpo-phalangeal pattern profiles in the evaluation of skeletal malformations. Radiology 104, 1—11 (1972)

18. POZNANSKI, A. K., GARN, S. M., SHAW, H. A.: The carpal angle in the congenital malformation syndromes. Ann. Radiol. 19, 141—150 (1976)

19. POZNANSKI, A. K., HOLT, J. F.: The carpals in congenital malformation syndromes. Am. J. Roentgenol. 112, 443—459 (1971)

20. POZNANSKI, A. K., MACPHERSON, R. I., GORLIN, R. J., GARN, S. M., NAGY, J. M., GALL, J. C. JR., STERN, A. M., DIJKMAN, D. J.: The hand in the oto-palato-digital syndrome. Ann. Radiol. 16, 203—209 (1973)

21. POZNANSKI, A. K.,   STEPHENSON, J. K.:   Radiographic findings in hypothalamic acceleration of growth associated with cerebral atrophy and mental retardation (cerebral gigantism). Radiology **88**, 446—456 (1967)

22. REEDER, M. M., FELSON, B.: Gamuts in Radiology. Cincinnati, Ohio: Audiovisual Radiology of Cincinnati, Inc. 1975

23. SINCLAIR, R. J. G., KITCHIN, A. H., TURNER, R. W. D.: The Marfan syndrome. Quarterly J. of Med. **53**, 19—46 (1960)

24. SLATER, S.: An evaluation of the metacarpal sign (short fourth metacarpal). Pediatrics **46** 468—471 (1970)

25. SMITH, D. W.: Recognizable Patterns of Human Malformation, 2nd ed. Philadelphia: W. B. Saunders 1976

26. SMITH, T. T.: A peculiarity in the shape of the hand in idiots of the "Mongol" type. Pediatrics **2**, 315—320 (1896)

27. WEAVER, D. D.,   GRAHAM, C. B.,   THOMAS, I. T., SMITH, D. W.: A new overgrowth syndrome with accelerated skeletal maturation, unusual facies, and camptodactyly. J. Pediatr. **84**, 547—552 (1974)

Lesions of the Spine

G. B. C. Harris

1. Introduction

Within the frame-work of this general title, I have chosen material to illustrate three points concerning the spine which I believe are of importance in pediatric radiology.

1. Congenital anomalies of the spine may be found in association with abnormalities in other organ systems, particularly with anomalies of foregut origin. For example, spine anomalies may be seen in association with gastrointestinal anomalies such as esophageal atresia, and with bronchopulmonary anomalies such as agenesis of a lung. I will show the value of the recognition of vertebral anomalies in helping to diagnose the presence of neuro-enteric anomalies.

2. Scoliosis may be the presenting complaint in a patient with a spinal cord tumor or with vertebral lesions such as osteoid osteoma or osteomyelitis. All too frequently such underlying causes of scoliosis are overlooked and appropriate therapy is delayed.

3. Persistent back pain in a child is a very important symptom. Unlike adults, backache in a child is almost always directly related to a significant underlying abnormality and requires thorough investigation. The radiologist must examine the films of the spine carefully for an underlying lesion such as infection, eosinophilic granuloma, tumor or trauma.

2. Vertebral Anomalies — a Useful Clue

Neuro-enteric anomalies are virtually always associated with congenital abnormalities in the formation and segmentation of some of the verte-brae. Various hypotheses have been put forth concerning the embryogenesis of this seemingly curious combination of intestinal anomalies connected to and associated with anomalies of the spine and its contents [1, 9]. They have in common the fact that at a very early stage of embryologic development the tissues destined to form the alimentary tract are physically close to ectodermal cells, which go on to form the spinal cord, and to the mesodermal tissues, which will form the vertebrae. Aberrations in formation of the enteric component may, therefore, be associated with anomalous development of the spine and its contents.

Patients with such neuro-enteric anomalies present with various abnormalities of the foregut including mediastinal enteric cyst, transdiaphragmatic intestinal duplication, anterior enteric diverticulum and right-sided congenital diaphragmatic hernia. The clue to the complete diagnosis is the presence of anomalies in the lower cervical and/or upper dorsal spine. The spectrum of spine anomalies varies from those which are quite gross and obvious, consisting of abnormalities in spinal segmentation with large defects in the vertebral bodies and widening of the neural canal (Fig. 1), through to lesser spine changes with small vertebral defects (Fig. 2) to even rather minor anomalies in segmentation (Fig. 3).

The importance of recognizing the spinal anomalies is illustrated by a 1-year-old girl who developed a few skin pustules which responded promptly to therapy. Shortly thereafter there was the onset of cough and fever. Radiographic examinations showed a right pleural effusion (Fig. 3a) and a presumptive diagnosis of pneumonia with empyema was made. She was treated with broad spectrum antibiotics and thoracocentesis was performed. Culture of the pleural fluid failed to grow

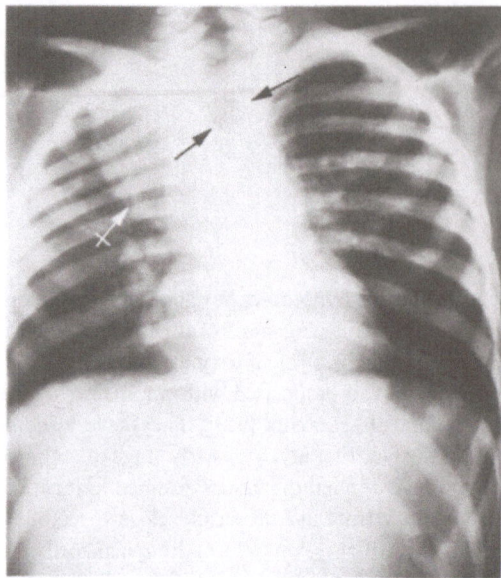

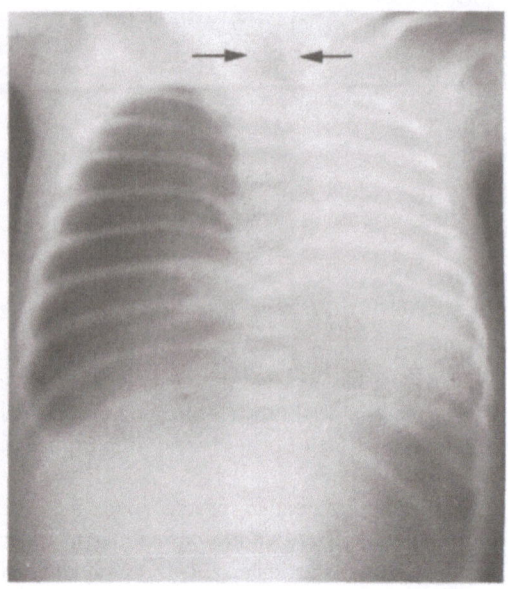

Fig. 1. Neuro-enteric malformation. Mediastinal enter-ogenous cyst(↔). Large and obvious defect in bodies of upper dorsal spine (→) indicates that this cyst is part of a neuroenteric malformation. A fibrous connection extended from cyst through spinal defect

Fig. 2. Neuro-enteric malformation. Appearance of right chest could be due to cystic malformation of lung. However, presence of rather minor vertebral body anomalies in lower cervical spine (→) provide clue that this is most likely a neuro-enteric malformation. This was a right diaphragmatic hernia with an anterior enteric diverticulum. Intestinal obstruction caused marked distention of bowel in the chest

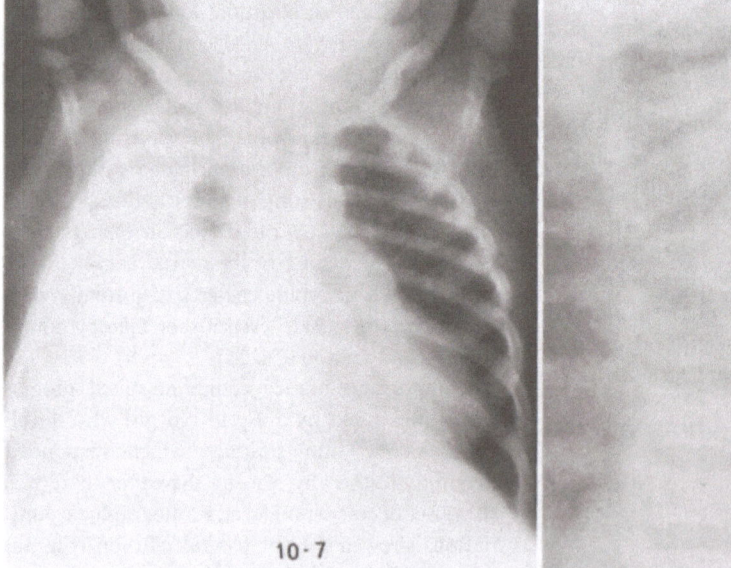

Fig. 3 a and b. Neuro-enteric malformation with minor spine anomaliex. a) First chest film showed a large pleural effusion which was mistakenly considered to be an empyema complicating an underlying pneumonia b) Minor upper dorsal spine anomalies were dismissed as being inconsequential. Weeks later, when the pleural effusion failed to improve, we placed more significance on the spine anomalies, leading us to the diagnosis of a neuroenteric malformation

any organisms, and the tuberculin test was negative. The pleural effusion recurred and the fever persisted. She was transferred to our hospital to evaluate the possibility of an underlying malignancy.

Little importance had initially been placed on the minor anomalies in the upper dorsal spine (Fig. 3 b). However, in view of the lack of clinical response to antibiotics, the negative pleural fluid culture and the finding of a high amylase level in the pleural fluid, the spine anomalies assumed greater significance. The possibility of a neuro-enteric anomaly with rupture into the pleural space was considered. Following further investigations, including examination of the upper gastrointestinal tract and an arteriographic study, exploratory surgery was done. This revealed a neuro-enteric diverticulum (Fig. 4) which extended from the pancreas up through the diaphragm along the dorsal spine to the lower cervical spine. In the lower right chest the diverticulum had a cystic dilatation which had ruptured into the pleural space which, in turn, caused the right-sided pleural effusion.

The case illustrates that in complex thoracic problems the presence of spine anomalies may provide a very useful clue leading to a better understanding of the patient's disorder.

3. Scoliosis as a Presenting Sign

Scoliosis is a comparatively common problem and it is most frequently of the so-called idiopathic type. It may also be found in association with congenital spinal anomalies, neuromuscular disorders, neurofibromatosis, congenital heart disease, etc.

The point I wish to emphasize is that scoliosis may be a presenting complaint in a patient in whom the underlying cause may be spinal cord tumor [11], or a vertebral lesion such as osteoid osteoma [3, 5] or infection. In such patients casual acceptance of the spinal curvature as simply another case of idiopathic scoliosis will result in potentially harmful delay in starting appropriate treatment. Spinal cord tumors are rare but, in a

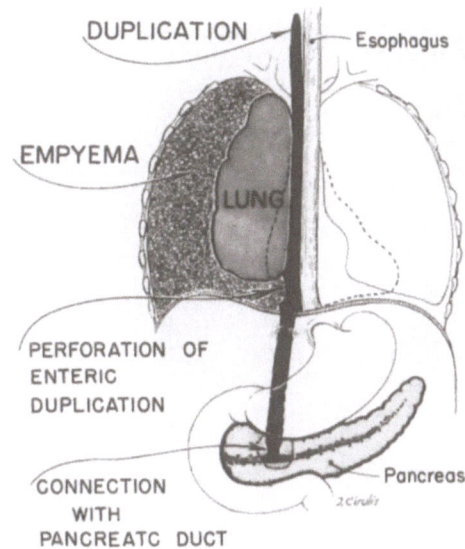

Fig. 4. Neuro-enteric malformation. Artist's rendition of anomaly found at operation. Perforation of neuro-enteric diverticulum allowed pancreatic secretions to enter right pleural space, resulting in reactive pleural effusion

large series, 27% of children with spinal cord tumors were found to have scoliosis [11]. In addition to scoliosis, there may be back pain, muscle spasm and weakness.

This problem is illustrated by the following boy who presented with a curvature of the spine at the age of four. He was considered to have idiopathic scoliosis and was treated for more than five years with back braces and exercises. On his radiographic examinations (Fig. 5) the widening of the neural canal was overlooked and the diagnosis of spinal cord astrocytoma was not made until 5 years later. It is important to radiograph the entire spine for, in some cases, while the scoliosis may be dorsal, the tumor may be in the cervical region. I advise our radiologists-in-training that when interpreting spine films of patients with scoliosis they should devote their time and attention to searching for possible causes of the scoliosis, and not concern themselves too much with measuring the degree of the curvature.

It should be remembered that scoliosis is not a diagnosis. Scoliosis should be considered as a physical sign, and where possible the cause should be identified.

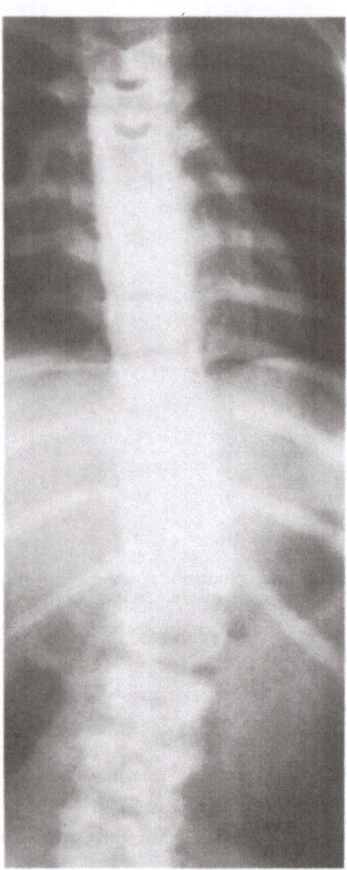

Fig. 5. Scoliosis—presenting sign of spinal cord tumor. Abnormally wide spinal canal in the lower dorsal spine went unnoticed for several years and the patient was treated for "idiopathic" scoliosis. Tumor of the cord was an astrocytoma

4. Back Pain in Children

Persistent or recurrent back pain in a child is a most important symptom and should never be neglected. Careful study will almost always uncover a definite cause. The causes of backache that are directly related to the spine include infection, eosinophilic granuloma, tumor and trauma.

4.1. Infection

Osteomyelitis of the spine usually causes fever and back pain. The pain may be referred to the abdomen or to the hip, and clinical attention may be diverted from the spine. The later radiographic signs are well known. Early in the disease, however, it may be quite difficult to recognize bone destruction on the plain films, due to superimposition of the overlying abdominal or thoracic viscera [10]. If there is any clinical suspicion of spinal osteomyelitis one must promptly resort to laminography and/or to the use of radioactive isotopes [6, 12]. The value of such studies is illustrated by the following patient, a teenage boy who presented with intermittent fever and pain in the mid-dorsal region. The plain films of the spine failed to reveal any abnormality, but when a radioactive isotope study was performed, it showed increased uptake in the mid-dorsal spine (Fig. 6). Laminography was then carried out, and showed a localized area of osteomyelitis in the vertebral body (Fig. 7). This proved to be a staphylococcal osteomyelitis, and the patient responded well to antibiotic treatment.

4.2. Eosinophilic Granuloma

Back pain is one of the cardinal signs of this disease when it involves the spine. Classically the radiographic appearance is one of vertebra plana with preservation of the adjacent intervertebral discs. The lesion, however, may at times involve the vertebral body in an asymmetric way [2] and may even extend into the pedicle (Fig. 8). With treatment the involved vertebra can be expected to undergo considerable reconstitution of its size and shape.

4.3. Tumors

Tumors of the vertebrae are almost always accompanied by back pain. Recognition of the lesion is usually not much of a problem since a good deal of destruction, expansion or distortion of the vertebral body or the arch has usually occurred by the time the patient presents. Among the tumors that may involve the spine in children are: aneurysmal bone cysts, osteoblastoma, osteoid osteoma and leukemia.

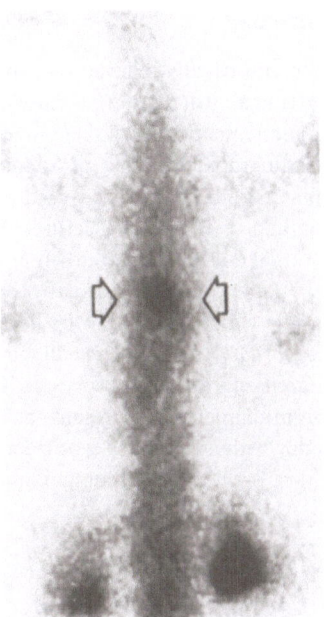

Fig. 6. Back pain—osteomyelitis. ^{99m}Tc bone scan shows increased activity in the mid-dorsal region

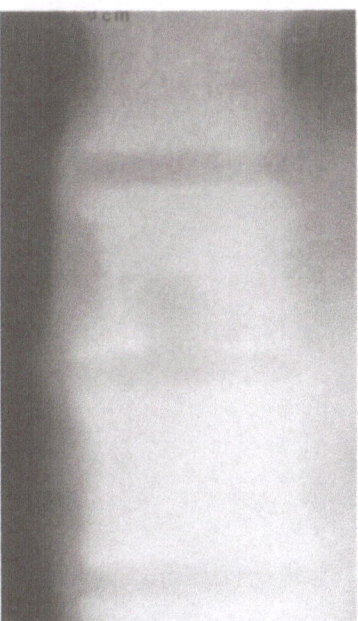

Fig. 7. Back pain—osteomyelitis. Subsequent laminogram shows small focus of destruction due to *Staphylococcal aureus* osteomyelitis. Plain films of this area were normal

4.4. Aneurysmal Bone Cyst

This is a fibrous tissue lesion, honeycombed with a dilated vascular network. In the spine it involves the neural arch and may expand into the body. Radiologically there is local rarefaction with expansion of the bone and thinning of the cortex to a thin egg-shell-like margin (Fig. 9).

4.5. Osteoblastoma

A benign tumor, this is sometimes called a giant osteoid osteoma [8]. It tends to be less painful than osteoid osteoma, producing a dull backache. Scoliosis occurs in about 30% of cases. The lesion usually involves the neural arch and pedicle with expansion of the bone (Fig. 10). It is usually lytic but generally has some calcification within its matrix. The size ranges from 1 to 10 cm. The surrounding margin of bone may be slightly sclerotic, but usually is less than that occurring with osteoid osteoma. Bone scan may be useful [7]. This lesion may be difficult to differentiate from aneurysmal bone cyst. Conservative surgical treatment is usually adequate.

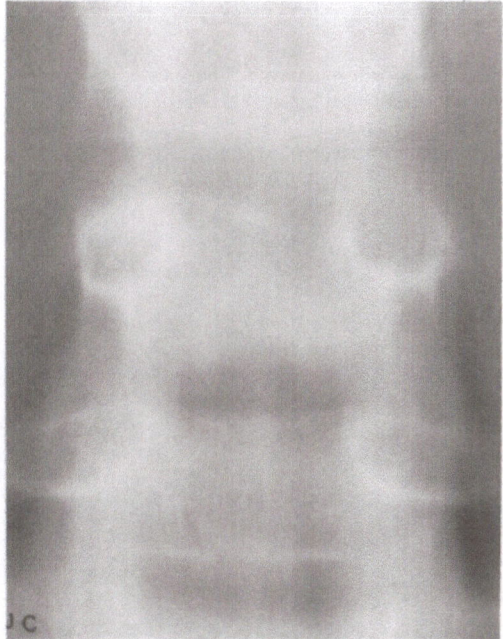

Fig. 8. Back pain—eosinophilic granuloma. This laminogram demonstrates destruction of the left superolateral portion of the body and of the adjacent pedicle. An unusual manifestation of eosinophilic granuloma. Radiation therapy was followed by excellent healing

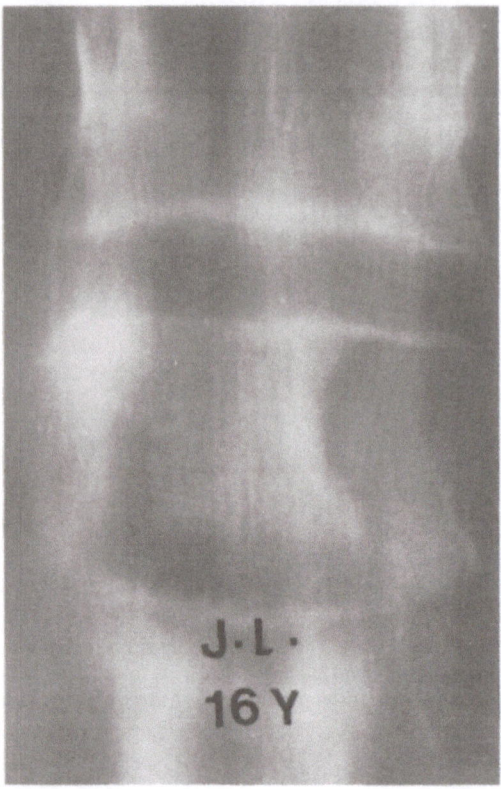

Fig. 9. Back pain—aneurysmal bone cyst. The lamino-gram reveals a localized area of lysis of the body and of the entire left pedicle. There was considerable expansion demonstrated on other films

4.6. Osteoid Osteoma

Pain, worse at night and usually relieved by aspirin, is an important and almost constant feature of osteoid osteoma. The patient may also have scoliosis [3, 5]. The radiographic changes of osteoid osteoma of the spine may be overlooked because of overlying abdominal or thoracic structures. It may be essential to make use of coned-down and oblique views, and laminography is usually required. Bone scanning with isotopes can be helpful in difficult cases [4]. The lesion usually involves the neural arch and articular processes. It is rarely over 1 cm in diameter and presents as a small zone of lucency with a central sclerotic density and with slightly sclerotic circumferential margins (Fig. 11).

4.7. Trauma

In a child presenting with back pain, one must also consider the possibility of trauma. Chronic or repetitive trauma or stress to the spine can result in a fatigue fracture of the neural arch. Trauma of this kind in children may occur in association with a variety of endeavors such as ballet dancing, gymnastics, hockey and other sports. The repetitive stress produces a fatigue fracture which is recognized as a defect in the region of the pars interarticularis [14]. If the fracture is not recognized

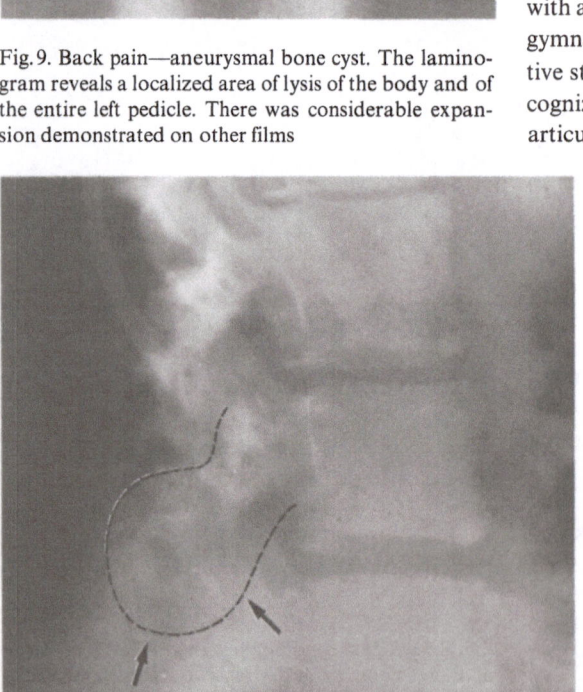

Fig. 10. Back pain—osteoblastoma. Marked expansion of posterior spinous process and neural arch. Matrix of tumor is calcified. Conservative surgical excision was followed by a good result

shortly after it occurs there is the likelihood of nonunion. Unilateral fatigue fracture of the pars interarticularis results in instability of the neural arch, and abnormal stresses are placed on the pedicle and neural arch of the side opposite to the fracture. The pedicle responds to the increased stresses with hypertrophy and sclerosis [13]. It is important to recognize this combination of uni-lateral fatigue fracture of the pars interarticularis with thickening and sclerosis of the contralateral pedicle (Fig. 12). Otherwise the dense, enlarged pedicle may be mistakenly diagnosed as being due to tumor, osteoid osteoma, or infection and inappropriate therapy may be instituted. Patients with this fracture should be treated by supportive braces and bedrest. If the pain and muscle spasm persists a spinal fusion may be necessary [13].

5. Summary

1. Congenital anomalies of the spine can be the key to recognizing neuro-enteric anomalies.
2. Scoliosis may be the presenting complaint in a child with a spinal cord tumor.

3. Back pain is an important complaint in a child. One must look carefully for osteomyelitis, eosino-philic granuloma, osteoid osteoma, tumor, leukemia or fatigue fracture.

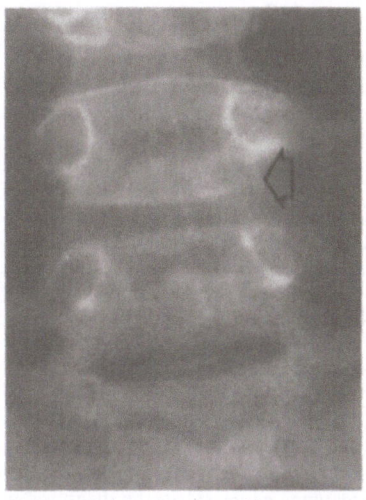

Fig. 11. Back pain—osteoid osteoma. Typical radio-graphic features are shown in this case. Small lytic area in the left side of the arch of L4. There is sclerosis of the surrounding bone and a small central density can be identified

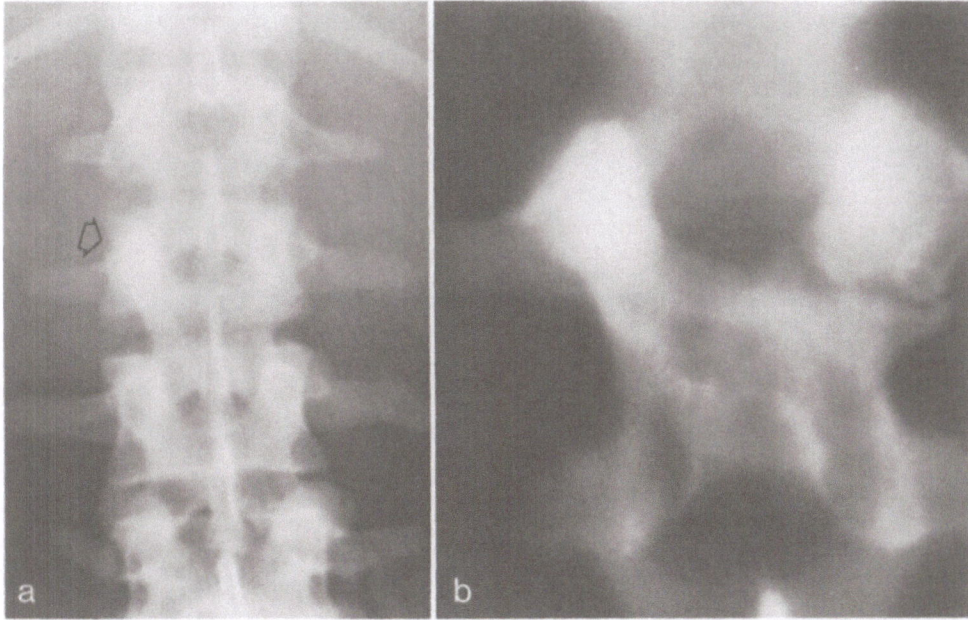

Fig. 12 a and b. Back pain—sclerotic pedicle—fractured pars. a) Young ballet dancer with back pain and slight lumbar scoliosis. Sclerotic right pedicle of L3 initially considered as possible osteoid osteoma

b) Laminogram shows fracture of pars interarticularis of left side of L3. Sclerosis of right pedicle due to reactive new bone formation secondary to abnormal stresses on neural arch because of the fracture

The roentgenographic investigation of backache in a child must be thorough, including laminography and radioactive bone scans.

References

1. BEARDMORE, H. E., WIGGLESWORTH, F. W.: Vertebral anomalies and alimentary duplications. Pediat. Clin. N. Amer. **5**, 457 (May 1958)
2. FERRIS, R. A., PETTRONE, F. A., McKELVIE, A. M., TWIGG, H. L., CHUN, B. K.: Eosinophilic granuloma of the spine: An unusual radiographic presentation. Clin. Orthop. **99**, 57 (1974)
3. FREIBERGER, R. H.: Osteoid osteoma of the spine. A cause of backache and scoliosis in children and young adults. Radiology **75**, 232 (1960)
4. GILDAY, D. L.: Diagnosis of obscure childhood osteoid osteomas with the bone scan. J. Nucl. Med. **15**, 494 (1974)
5. KEIM, H. A., REINA, E. G.: Osteoid osteoma as a cause of scoliosis. J. Bone Jt. Surg. **57 A**, 159 (1975)
6. LETTS, R. M., AFITI, A., SUTHERLAND, J. B.: Technetium bone scanning as an aid in the diagnosis of atypical osteomyelitis in children. Surg. Gynec. Obstet. **140**, 899 (1975)
7. MARTIN, N. L., PRESTON, D. F., ROBINSON, R. G.: Osteoblastomas of the axial skeleton shown by skeletal scanning, Case report. J. Nucl. Med. **17**, 187 (1976)
8. McLEOD, R. A., DAHLIN, D. C., BEABOUT, J. W.: The spectrum of osteoblastoma. Amer. J. Roentgenol. **126**, 321 (1976)
9. MILLS, R. R., HOLMES, A. E.: Enterogenous cyst of the spinal cord with associated intestinal reduplication, vertebral anomalies and a dorsal dermal sinus. J. Neurosurg. **38**, 73 (1973)
10. MUSHER, D. M., THORSTEINSSON, S. B., MINUTH, J. N., LUCHI, R. J.: Vertebral osteomyelitis—still a diagnostic pitfall. Arch. intern. Med. **136**, 105 (1976)
11. TACHDJIAN, M. O., MATSON, D. D.: Orthpaedic aspects of intraspinal tumors in infants and children. J. Bone Jt. Surg. **47 A**, 230 (1965)
12. TREVES, S., KHETTRY, F. H., BROKER, F. H., WILKINSON, R. H., WATTS, H.: Osteomyelitis: Early Scintigraphic detection in children. Pediatrics **57**, 173 (1976)
13. WILKINSON, R. H., HALL, J. E.: The sclerotic pedicle: tumor or pseudo-tumor? Radiology **111**, 683 (1974)
14. WILTSE, L. L., WIDELL, E. H., JACKSON, D. W.: Fatigue fracture: the basic in isthmic spondylolisthesis. J. Bone Jt. Surg. **57 A**, 17 (1975)

Hydrocephalus in Children. A Radiological Study

M. Hassan

1. Definition and Classification

Hydrocephalus generally refers to a group of conditions associated with ventricular enlargement and the presence of an increased quantity of cerebrospinal fluid (CSF) under increased pressure, the latter being present either intermittently or persistently, now or sometime in the past. Hydrocephalus associated with a tumoral obstruction is not included in this paper, because in these cases the clinical picture is generally completely different, and consequently the radiologic approach differs. Only some of the difficulties which can arise will be discussed in the differential diagnosis. Ventricular enlargement due to primary atrophic or hypoplastic cerebral conditions is not related to pressure changes, and thus should not be included in a study of hydrocephalus. In these disorders, the primary site of the disease is in the substance of the brain, with enlargement of the ventricles occuring passively and secondarily.

Hydrocephalus in children results from an obstruction at some point along the CSF pathways. According to BELL and MACCORMICK [1] it is convenient to classify hydrocephalus as:

1. Intraventricular obstructive hydrocephalus (IVO), formerly called noncommunicating. This variety is most likely to occur because of abnormalities in areas where the pathways are narrow, including the aqueduct of Sylvius, the fourth ventricle and the foramen of Monro.

2. Extraventricular obstructive hydrocephalus (EVO), formerly named communicating. It is related to an obstruction at some point distal to the outlet formania of the fourth ventricle, usually at the level of the basilar cisterns, or within the arachnoid over the surface of the brain, or at the presumed absorptive site, the arachnoid villi.

2. Distribution of Patients

In our series, EVO accounts for 57.5% of the patients. In 20.5% of the remaining cases we found aqueduct abnormalities. Hydrocephalus was associated with myelomeningocele in 10% of the patients, and with Dandy-Walker malformation in 9%. Finally there were 6 cases (3%) of Choroid plexus papillomas. Most of the patients (68%) of our series are below 6 months of age and 82% are less than a year old. For most of them the clinical problem has been very simple: an infant with an enlarging head.

3. Plain Skull Examination

Changes on plain films are obvious in most of the hydrocephalic patients, as has been stated by SCHEY [17]. These findings can be separated into two groups:

a) Changes related to the hydrocephalic state no matter what the cause: in this group there is an absolute enlargement of the skull which can be demonstrated by measurements. It is more convenient to appreciate the exaggerated craniofacial disproportion of the infant on the lateral view (Fig. 1). The degree of bulging of the anterior fontanel can be easily appreciated on a lateral view of the skull, when subjected to bright light observation. This sign is influenced neither by the child's position during the radiographic procedure nor by whether the child is crying or not. During the first month there are considerable variations in the sutural width in healthy babies, and the degree of sutural diastasis is difficult to evaluate. The

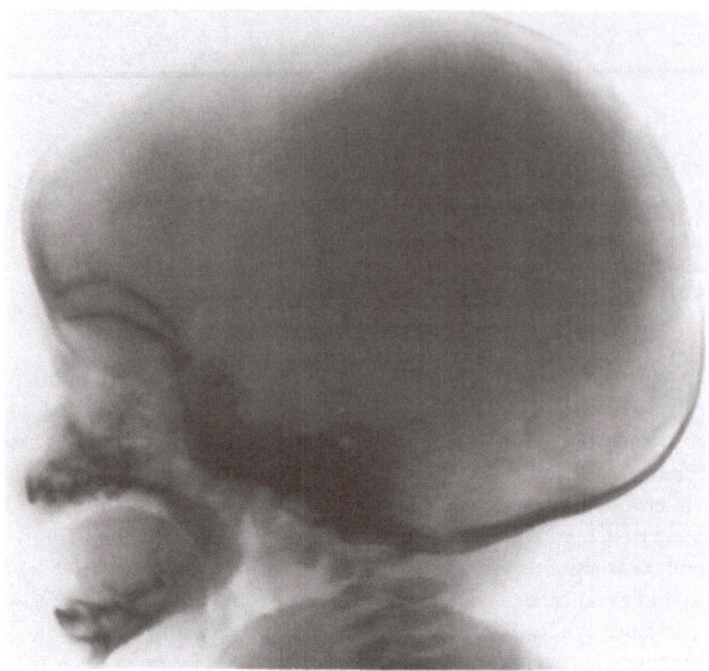

Fig. 1. Hydrocephalus with aqueduct stenosis (2 months). Plain skull film: note the exaggerated craniofacial disproportion. Posterior fossa index is rather small. Sutures are large and wide

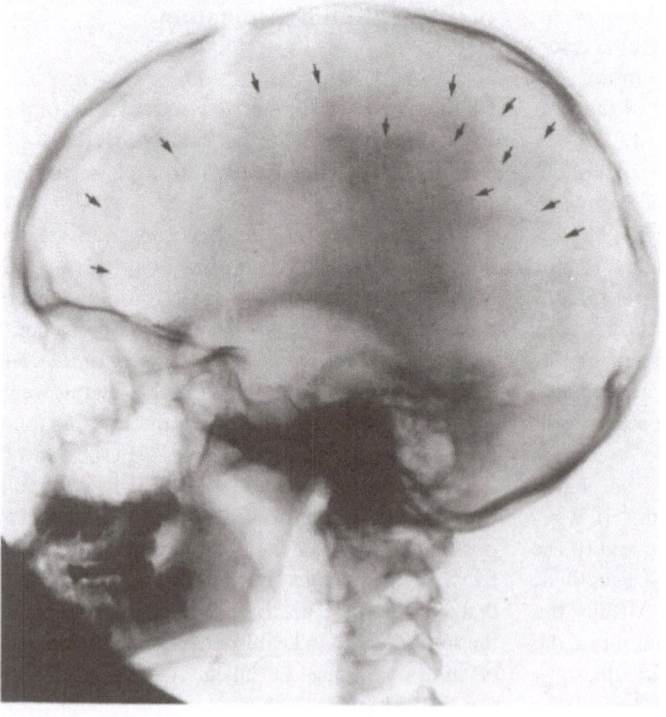

Fig. 2. Hydrocephalus by aqueductal stenosis in an 11-year-old girl. Note in this case the classical skull changes of intracranial hypertension (sutures, sella turcica). There are small and numerous punctate calcifications (arrow) around the dilated lateral ventricles. These are suggestive of toxoplasmosis

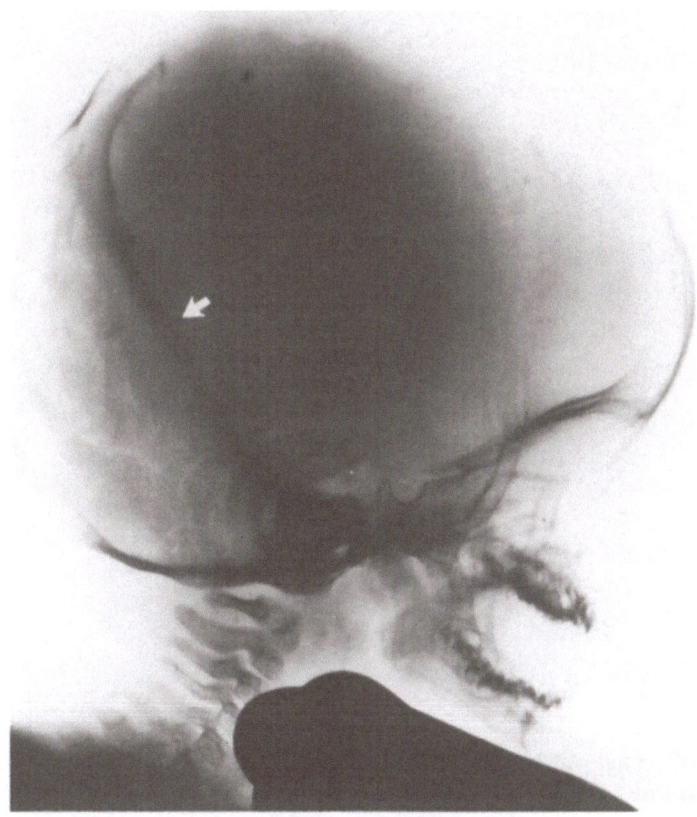

Fig. 3. Dandy-Walker syndrome (1-year-old boy). Plain skull examination. Note elevated position of lateral sinus grooves *(arrow)* which is pathognomonic, but not constant in this syndrome

splitting of the sutures, however, is an excellent sign in older children (Fig. 2). Less significant are the degree of thinness of the parietal bones, frontal bossing, bathrocephaly, and finally the state of the sella and clinoids particularly in the case of the infant and young child.

b) Changes more or less specific for various etiologies: The size of the posterior fossa must be evaluated. For this, SCHEY's posterior fossa index seems very suitable [17]. A very small index is suggestive of an aqueductal obstruction. Asymmetry of the skull, with or without local thinning, must be looked for, as it is suggestive of an associated cyst. In the Dandy-Walker cyst, the skull hypertrophy tends to predominate posteriorly (Fig. 3). Further more, in the Dandy-Walker anomaly, it must be stressed that the classic findings, such as the elevated lateral sinus grooves, are not often noticed on the plain films before 4 or 5 years of age. Craniolacunae (or Lückenschädel) is

quite pathognomonic of Arnold Chiari malformation associated with myelomeningocele. Craniolacunae, of course, must be distinguished from the beaten silver appearence: generally the first patterns disappear by 8–12 months of age, while digital markings are not visualized before 3 years of age. In patients with myelomeningocele YU and DUCK [22] have reported an obvious deformity of the basiocciput: marked concavity clearly restricted to the basiocciput, with extreme thinning of the bone (Fig. 6). It is a very frequent finding, probably due to local pressure from the pons in a narrowed posterior fossa.

Intracranial calcifications can be observed. Linear or spotted, they often follow the outline of the lateral ventricles (Fig. 2) or are located around the foramen of Monro. They are strongly suggestive of congenital toxoplasmosis.

Finally, although the plain skull study is very often helpful, in a few cases, the hydrocephalic skull

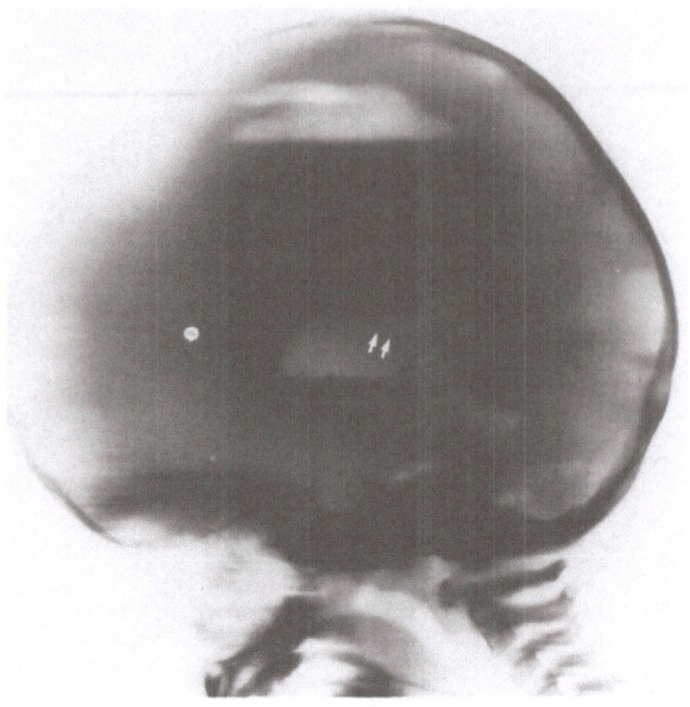

Fig. 4. IVO hydrocephalus associated with suprasellar cyst examined by pneumoencephalography (midline tomography). Note shape of sella turcica: very suggestive of a cyst. Cyst is fitted from the basilar cisterns, and pushes third ventricle upward. Membrane of cyst is well demonstrated (*arrow*)

radiograph can be somewhat confusing. This is the case especially in older children in whom hydrocephalus has been well compensated up to now. The appearance is that of intracranial hypertension, often mimicking a posterior fossa tumor. Sellar changes are obvious; also, digital markings are impressively increased, with tremendous splitting of sutures (Fig. 2). The rare cases of so-called normal pressure hydrocephalus (NPH) can also be confusing: the vault is somewhat enlarged, but there is no evidence of intracranial pressure despite the advanced age of the patient (Fig. 5).

4. Special Procedures and Results

Two methods have prevailed until now in the radiological approach to the diagnosis of hydrocephalus: arterial and ventricular (air or/and positive contrast) studies. In recent times the advent of CAT computerized tomography (CT) has completely changed the philosophy of neuroradiologic work. Our own experience of C.T. is rather limited as yet but ventricular enlargement is quickly and beautifully demonstrated by CT.

Some authors have published their first results with CT in hydrocephalus [12]. However, no definite statement can yet, be given as regards the upholding or the exclusion of conventionnal methods in the current evaluation of hydrocephalus. Furthermore, the pathology does not differ, whatever becomes of X-ray machines. Angiography has been put forward by RAIMONDI [14] and by CASTAN [4] as the mandatory method for evaluating hydrocephalus. However, many authors, and it is also our personal opinion, consider that the best way to appreciate the true morphology of the ventricles and the site and form of the obstruction, is indeed to deal directly with these structures. Furthermore, we consider that, in very young infants, air or positive contrast studies are generally safer than angiographic procedures. For these reasons our approach has been essentially a ventricular one, with pneumoencephalography and/or positive contrast ventriculography as the first and very often the only step. Except in particuliar cases, the study is usually begun with a pneumoencephalography. If a block is encountered, we then perform a ventricular tap and ventriculography during the same procedure. We have been using, for the past five years, a water soluble contrast medium, the Dimer X [7]. Nowadays it will be more convenient to use Metrizamide as it has been shown to be a safer contrast medium for brain studies.

EVO Hydrocephalus. This variety is characterized by a free ventricular pathway. The air injected by lumbar puncture can progress to the entire ventricular system. Typically there is a dilatation of the lateral, the third, and the fourth ventricles. The latter is generally proportionally less dilated. The third and fourth ventricles are not displaced. The dilatation of the lateral ventricles is usually symmetrical, sometimes asymmetrical. Commonly, this procedure can demonstrate a block at the level of the basilar cisterns (Fig. 5). This block is generally considered as a true reflection of the primary pathology of the disease. However, it has been stated [14] that such an appearence can be produced by a dilated third ventricle, even if the basilar cisterns are anatomically normal. Nevertheless, when such a pattern is observed with sufficient air injected, a basal block can be assumed. It must be stressed that the degree of the dilatation of the lateral ventricles does not directly correlate with the adverse effects of hydrocephalus in respect of mental development in particular, except in extreme cases. For follow-up evaluation and reporting, it is convenient to measure the dilatation, either by measuring the distance, in the lateral brow-up position, from the diploë to the anterior horn [3], or by the EVANS ratio [5] which is also reliable. SHURTLEFF [18] has elaborated a "formula" which allows him to correlate the "brain mass" to the DQ-IQ evolution after shunting.

Some abnormalities may be associated with EVO hydrocephalus and some of them act as determinants for poor prognosis: they include porencephalic cysts generally communicating with the ventricles and midline abnormalities such as septal cysts, leakage of the septum and corpus callosum dysgenesis. The most interesting are the arachnoid abnormalities associated with EVO hydrocephalus [2]. Not uncommonly, very huge pouches are encountered located within the arachnoid: suprasellar cysts, cisterna magna cysts or quadrigeminal plate cysts. Suprasellar cysts communicate with the basal cisterns. They often compress the third ventricle upward [13]. In one of our case (Fig. 4) the changes in the sella were quite similar to those which occur in the Hurler-Hunter syndrome. Cisterna magna cysts may compress the fourth ventricle forward, and during pneumoencephalography this cavity may not fill in the usual sitting position. These cysts do not go down below the foramen magnum, as do the Dandy-Walker cysts. Quadrigeminal cysts or venae magnae cerebri cisterna cysts may occur, and tend to extend within the roof of the third ventricle. They must be differentiated from cystic pinealomas.

In this group of EVO hydrocephalus associated with myelomeningocele must be studied. There is a free pathway through the ventricular system, although the course is somewhat extended. The exact mechanism of the hydrocephalus in this disease is not clear. The typical pattern can be demonstrated in most of the patients by ventriculography which provides very good visualization (Fig. 6). There is a caudal herniation of the cerebellum, tonsils, brainstem, and fourth ventricle into the upper cervical canal. These changes are described as ARNOLD CHIARI malformation type II. There are a lot of developmental anomalies of the brain and its covering. Some of them may be demonstrated. Such are the changes in the third ventricle [8] which include coronal transventricular connexus inferior to the anterior commissure, pseudo diverticulum through the lamina terminalis, enlarged massa intermedia and supplementary diverticulum in the posterior aspect of the third ventricle. Hydromelia can also be encountered at times.

To complete this chapter on EVO hydrocephalus we must mention three special entities. First, the rare cases of hydrocephalus related to impaired venous drainage of CSF. Such hydrocephalus may be observed in superior vena caval obstruction, and we have seen the development of hydrocephalus after a Mustard operation for transposition of the great vessels. Secondly there are the cases associated with foramen magnum abnormalites: the most common is hydrocephalus

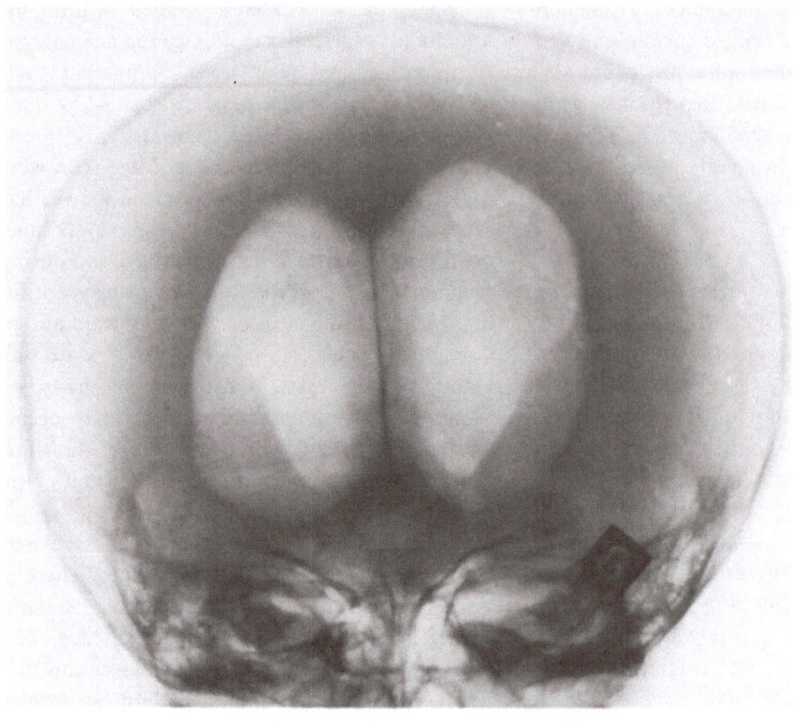

Fig. 5a.

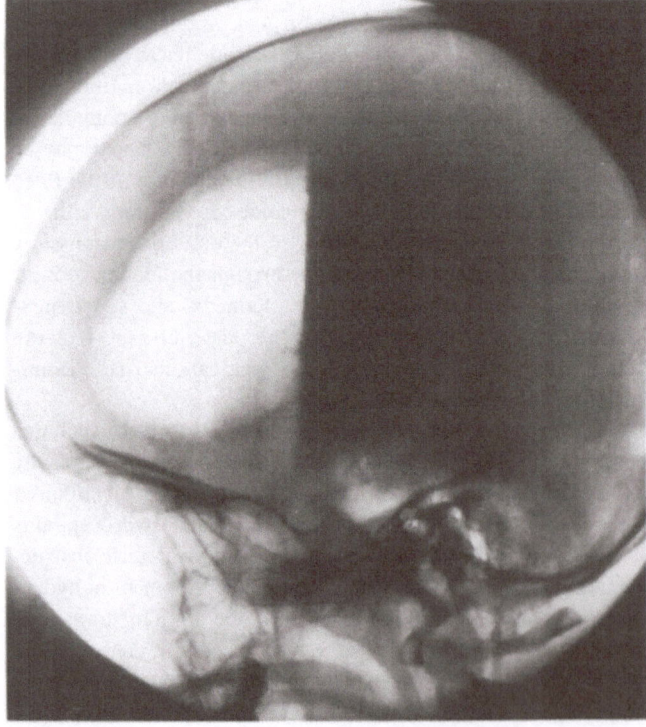

Fig. 5b.

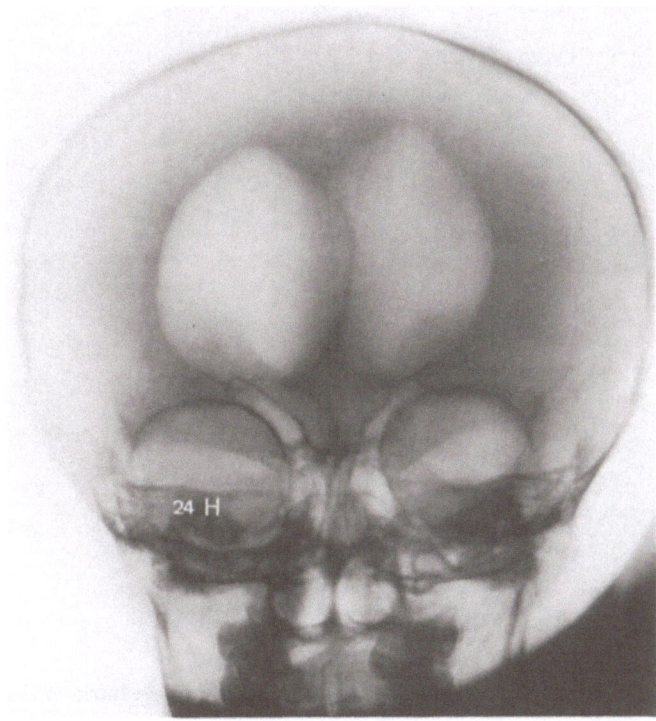

Fig. 5c.

Fig. 5 a—c. NPH hydrocephalus in an 8-year-old girl, examined by pneumoencephalography. Lateral ventricles are considerably dilated. There is a block at the basilar system. Note that there is no evidence of ele- vated intracranial pressure on the skull film. Twenty four hours after the examination (c) air remains and septum is bowed. This examination considerably worsened the clinical state of the patient

Fig. 6. Hydrocephalus associated with spina bifida. Water-soluble ventriculography. Typical appearance with caudal herniation of fourth ventricle and tonsils (arrow). Note pseudodiverticulum in posterior aspect of third ventricle (arrow head). There is also a coronal transventricular nexus (line). Note marked concavity of basiocciput and extreme thinning of bone

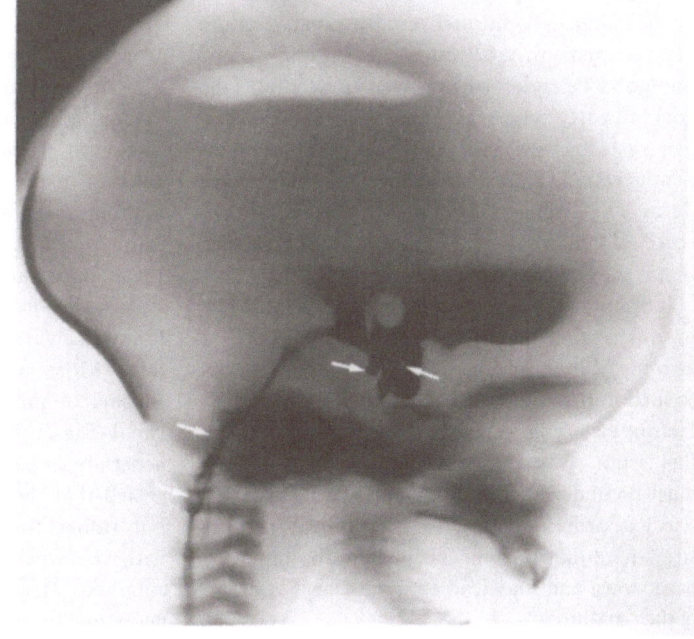

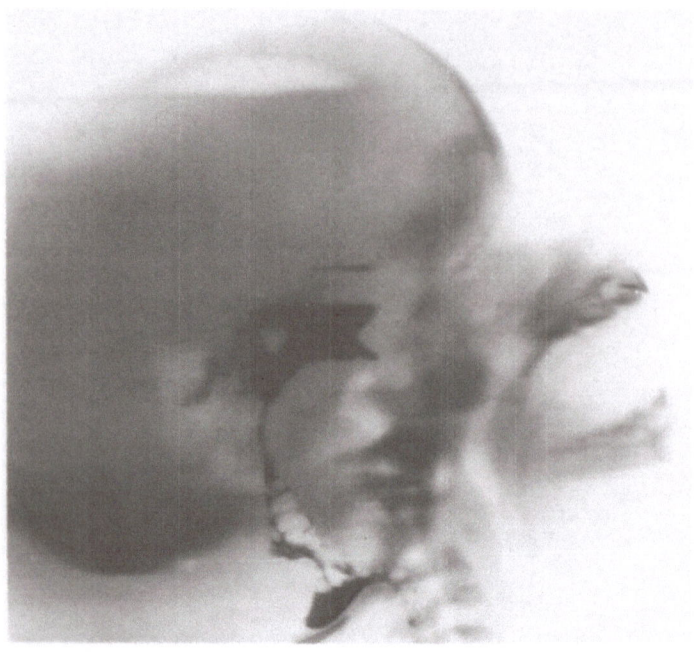

Fig. 7. Aqueduct stenosis (4 months). Combined pneumoencephalography and water-soluble ventriculography. Extreme narrowing of aqueduct. Contrast medium nevertheless passes through the aqueduct

which occurs in achondroplastic patients and although the exact mechanism is not clear, it is generally thought that it is a consequence of flow impairment in a narrowed foramen magnum.

The third entity which much be discussed here is the so called normal pressure hydrocephalus (NPH) [10, 21] (Fig. 5). Features of NPH include ventriculomegaly, normal cerebrospinal pressure at measurement, intellectual retardation, a curious good behavior pattern well designated "the cocktail party syndrome", neurologic deficiencies, gait disturbances, and finally favourable therapeutic response to ventricular shunting procedures. The diagnosis is difficult because of the absence of the main criterion for hydrocephalus, that is the enlarging head, or at least skull changes of intracranial hypertension. The main problem is to differentiate accurately NPH from cortical atrophy. None of the radiologic findings described in the adult cases is pathognomonic [21]. Isotope cisternography may be of importance, but this is not always the case. Many investigations must be undertaken in these patients in order to select appropriate cases for shunting. We must stress here that pneumoencephalography may be hazardous, and may lead to a sudden worsening of the condition.

Intraventricular Obstruction (IVO). Here, diagrammatically a dilatation of the cavities located above the block is observed, while those situated below it remain normal.

The more common are the aqueduct abnormalities. Most of them are considered to be congenital. RUSSELL [15] has classified the lesions from a neuropathological point of view as gliosis, forking, true narrowing and a septum. SCHECHTER and ZUNGESSER [16] have attempted to classify the radiographic appearance of the stenosed aqueduct into six types, but there was considerable overlap in the roentgen appearance. The use of combined water soluble ventriculography and lumbar air injection provides a good approach to these abnormalities. With such an approach it has become less frequent to observe a complete block followed by a dilated initial portion of the aqueduct. More often the contrast medium passes through a more or less regular but narrowed canal (Fig. 7). The fourth ventricle is midline and generally small. WILLIAMS [20] has recently suggested that the stenosis was not truly the cause, but rather the consequence of hydrocephalus, with a compression of the midbrain caused by the enlarged lateral ventricles. Further studies are necessary to clarify this problem, but at present

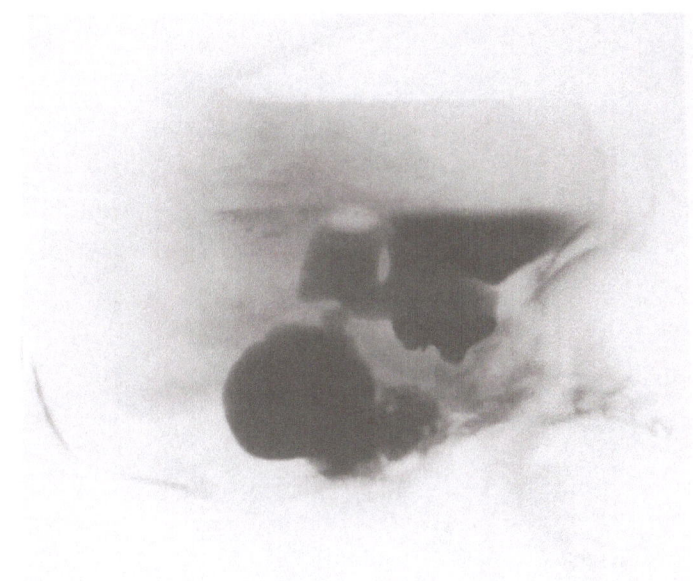

Fig. 8. IVO hydrocephalus from obstruction of Magendie and Luschka foramina. Water-soluble ventriculography. Fourth ventricle is huge, but still recognizable. Contrast medium does not progress below the foramen magnum

most people think that genuine cases of primary aqueduct disturbances do obviously exist. In such hydrocephalus, a sex-linked disease must be suspected in every male patient [9] even if there is not the "typical appearence" reported by ED-WARDS, namely, the maldevelopment of the thumbs (flexus adductus).

Obstruction beneath the fourth ventricle represents another important cause of hydrocephalus. There are two forms: the congenital one, known as the Dandy-Walker syndrom and the acquired one secondary to presumed adhesive archnoiditis in the posterior fossa. In acquired occlusion of the MAGENDIE and LUSHKA foramina, a huge fourth ventricle is demonstrated, but the cavity is still recognizable. The contrast medium does not reach either the cervical canal or the posterior fossa cisterns (Fig. 8).

The Dandy-Walker malformation is more complex. The presumed cause is an early closure during fetal life of the fourth ventricle foramina, resulting in a cystic transformation of this cavity with a disproportionate increase in size of the posterior fossa. The vermis is absent or hypoplastic. Other anomalies may coexist. Typically, the cyst is not filled by air injected by the lumbar route; however, at times, this can occur. When the diag-

nosis is suspected, vertebral angiography can be useful (Fig. 9). It will demonstrate a lateral displacement of the posterior cerebral arteries; these vessels do not approach the midline as they pass over the surface of the occipital lobes. On the lateral view, the posterior cerebral arteries are considerably elevated, and on the venous phase the straight sinus is seen in a very high position. Ventriculography clearly shows the cystic feature to be very extensive. The cavity generally passes through the foramen magnum into the upper cervical canal. The Dandy-Walker cyst is often associated with cervical meningocele, that is with Arnold Chiari type III malformation.

IVO can also occur above the fourth ventricle and especially in the foramen of Monro. It may be bilateral or unilateral, causing an asymmetrical hydrocephalus. In this group of IVO one must also discuss vascular malformations, especially the aneurysm of the vein of Galen. Attention is alerted when there is a definite bruit heard over the head or when there is heart failure. Cerebral angiography is then mandatory, and it readily demonstrates the huge malformation with numerous feeding arteries and considerable dilatation of the Galenic system (Fig. 10). At times, the diagnosis is not suspected clinically: it may be suggested

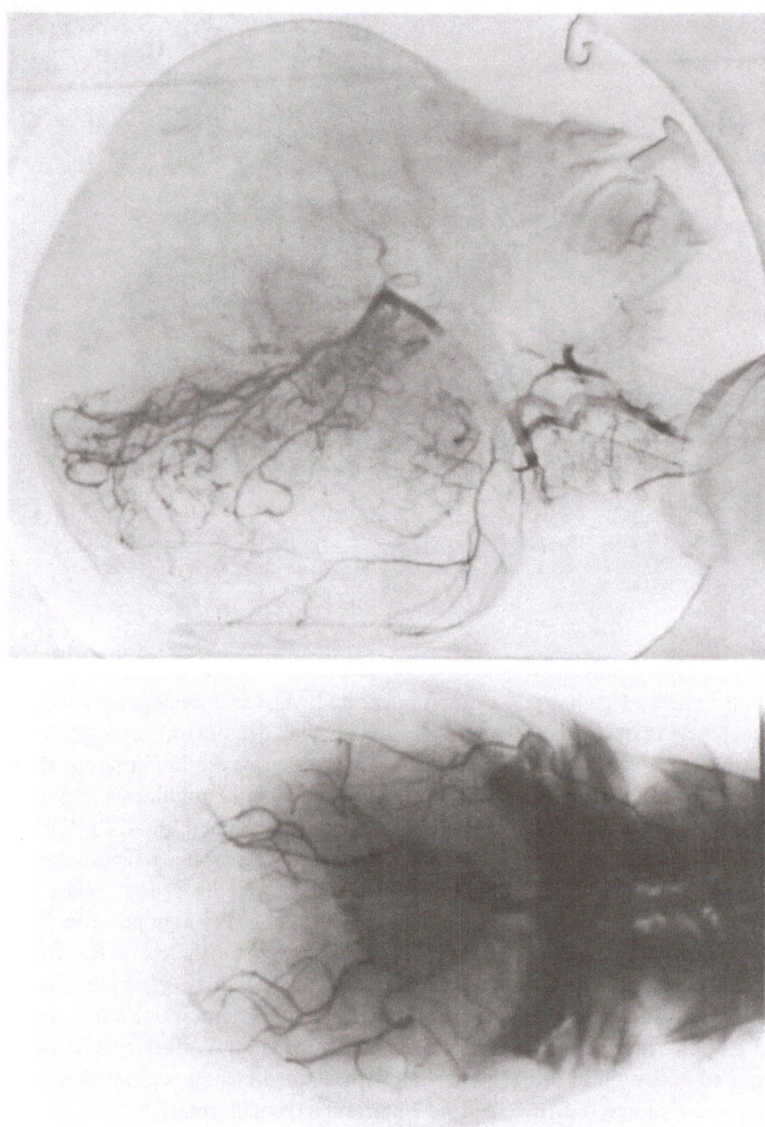

Fig. 9a and b. Dandy-Walker syndrome (1 year). Vertebral angiography, arterial phase. Typical appearance: elevated cerebral posterior arteries; these vessels do not approach midline on frontal projection

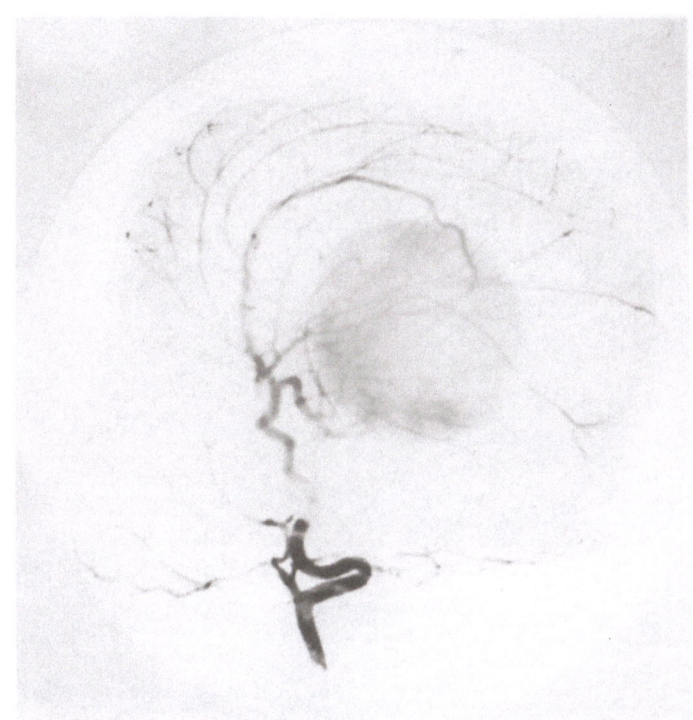

Fig. 10. Hydrocephalus with aneurysm of the vein of Galen (5 months). Carotid arteriography demonstrates, associated with hydrocephalus the huge aneurysm of Galen vein. The malformation is opacified very soon and by numerous feeding vessels

when the appearance of the aqueduct is irregular or when there is a mass effect on the posterior aspect of the third ventricle.

Plexus Choroid Papillomas (PCP). These tumors are responsible for a peculiar form of hydrocephalus. Clinically, the diagnosis can at times be suspected because of the very high protein content of the CSF. Isotope scanning may also suggests PCP. Nevertheless, the true diagnosis is often made on radiologic examination. Hydrocephalus, secondary to PCP, is generally asymmetric and nonobstructive. It must be stressed that sufficient air is necessary to give a good demonstration of the tumor because this tumor is often pedunculated and may be hidden by the fluid in the ventricles. PCP arise more often in the trigone area (Fig. 11), but also in the third and the fourth ventricles. They may be benign or malignant. Very often multiple investigations [19] are necessary to ascertain the diagnosis. Angiography is most valuable, since these tumors are usually highly vascular. They are supplied by the choroidal arteries, anterior and/or posterior.

5. Differential Diagnosis

There are in fact only a few differential diagnoses. However, some errors must be avoided. Some enlarged heads are not related to hydrocephalus; they may or may not be familial, but generally a close follow-up of the cranial perimeter is sufficient. Sometimes neuroradiologic work-up is necessary: CT will be most helpful in these cases.

Hydrocephalus must be differenciated from cerebral atrophy: typically in atrophy, there is a rounding of the margins of the lateral ventricles, and in the frontal brow up position, the callosum angle [21] is greater than 140°; also, air is present in large amount intra cranially, and on the angiogram the vessels are not stretched. None of these criteria is absolutely cardinal, and at times the distinction is not possible on the ventricular pattern alone. We consider that the most reliable sign is the absence of an enlarging head or intracranial hypertension in such cases of brain atrophy.

The problem is somewhat more complex when NPH is considered: we have carefully studied

a)

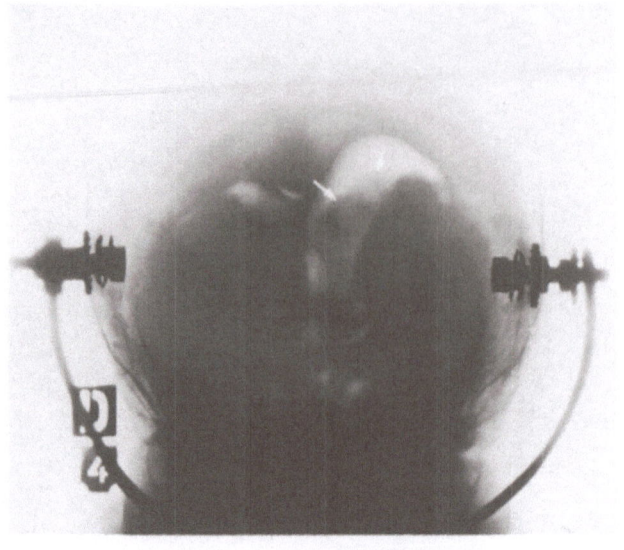

b)

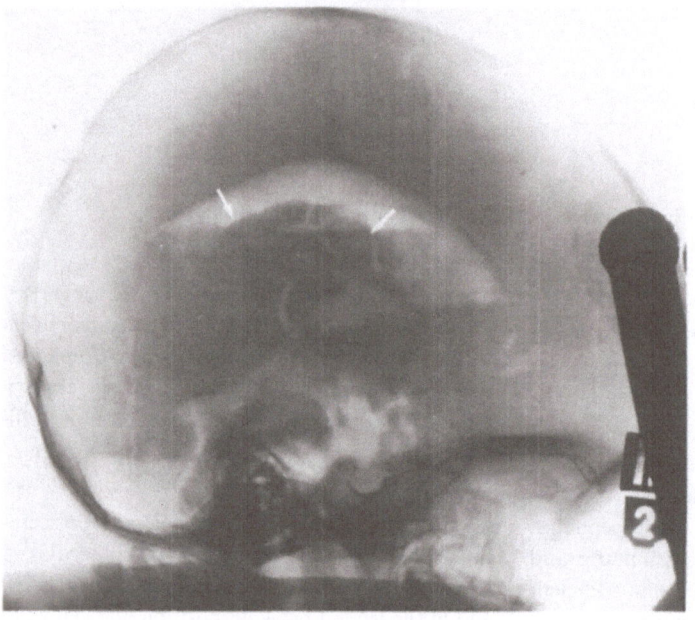

Fig. 11 a and b. Plexus choroid papilloma of the trigone area. Pneumoencephalography: there is an asymmetrical hydrocephalus. The papilloma is visible inside lateral ventricle (*arrow*), with a typical cauliflower appearence

these rare cases. The main problems arise in older children. One must be careful when the clinical history is not suggestive; that is, when there has not been a progressive enlargement of the head since birth or when there is no positive history of meningeal disturbances.

When posterior fossa tumors are being considered the problem is easy to solve: symptoms rarely fail to suggest the diagnosis and ventriculography will always demonstrate the lesions. The case is more difficult when the neuroradiologic pattern is that of an EVO without supporting clinical features. The diagnosis of "idiopathic EVO" hydrocephalus must not be easily accepted. Spinal tumors must be looked for; they may produce hydrocephalus. Elsewhere, only follow-up studies may discover the real cause of the disease, as in meningeal malignancy or intracranial tumors not visible on the first examination.

6. Conclusion

Hydrocephalus in children mostly occurs during the first year of life. The positive diagnosis is usually easy on clinical and purely radiologic grounds. Neuroradiologic work-up is necessary to ascertain the diagnosis, to evaluate the degree of ventricular enlargment, and to assess the site and type of the block. It is possible that in the near future C.T. will be sufficient in most cases as the only step before shunting.

References

1. BELL, W. E., McCORMICK, W. F.: Increased Intra Cranial Pressure in Children. In: Major Problems in Clinical Pediatrics, Saunders 1972, Vol. VIII
2. BERKMEN, Y. M., BRUCHER, J., SALMON, J. H.: Congenital arachnoid cysts. Amer. J. Roentgen-Rad. Therap. Nucl. Med. **105**, 2, 298—304 (1969)
3. BURHENNE, H. J., DAVIES, H.: The ventricular span in cerebral pneumography. Amer. J. Roentgen. **90**, 1176—1184 (1963)
4. CASTAN, P., BOUZIGE, J. C., CASTAN-TARBOUR-EICH, E.: Les hydrocephalies de l'enfant. Angiographie cérébrale 1975, Expansion Scientifique publisher (Paris), 1 vol.
5. EVANS, W. A.: An encephalographic ratio for estimating the size of the cerebral ventricles. Amer. J. dis. child. **64**, 820—830 (1942)
6. GILLES, F. H., SHILLITO, J. JR.: Infantile hydrocephalus retrocerebellar subdural hematoma. J. Pediat. **76**, 529—537 (1970)
7. GONSETTE, R.: An experimental and clinical assessment of water-soluble contrast medium in neuroradiology. A new medium: Dimer X. Clin. Radiol. **22**, 44—56 (1971)
8. GOODING, C. A., CARTER, A., HOARE, R. D.: New ventriculographic aspects of the Arnold Chiari malformation. Radiology **89**, 626—632 (1967)
9. HOLMES, L. B., NASH, A., ZURHEIN, G., LEVIN, M., OPITZ, J.: X-linked aqueduct stenosis. Clinical and neurophathological findings in two families. Pediatrics **51**, 697—704 (1973)
10. MILHORAT, T. H., HAMMOCK, M. K.: "Arrested" versus normal pressure hydrocephalus in children. Clin. Proc. children's hospital National Medical Center **28**, 168—173 (1972)
11. MILHORAT, T. H.: Hydrocephalus and the CSF. Baltimore (Maryland): Williams & Wilkins 1972
12. NAICICH, T. P., EPSTEIN, F., LIN, J. P., KRICHEFF, I. J., HOCHWALD, G. M.: Evaluation of pediatric hydrocephalus by computed tomography. Radiology **119**, 337—345 (1976)
13. PIERRE-KAHN, A., SACHS, M., HIRSCH, J. F.: Hydrocephalie et kyste arachnoidien supra sellaire. Neurochirurgie **20**, 179—190 (1974)
14. RAIMONDI, A. J.: Hydrocephalus in Pediatric Neuroradiology. 1972, Saunders Co. publishers, pp. 147—389
15. RUSSEL, D. S.: Observations on the pathology of hydrocephalus. Spec. Rep. Ser. med. Res. Coun. n 1949, No. 265
16. SCHECHTER, M. M., ZINGESSER, L. H.: The radiology of aqueductal stenosis. Radiology **88**, 905 (1967)
17. SCHEY, W.: Plain film skull roentgenographic changes in hydrocephalus. Amer. J. Roentgenol. Radiol. Thera. Nucl. Med. **118**, 134—146 (1973)
18. SHURTLEFF, D. B., FOLTZ, E. L., LOESER, J. D.: Hydrocephalus: a definition of its progression and relationship to intellectual function, diagnosis and complication. Am. J. Dis. Child. **125**, 688—693 (1973)
19. THOMPSON, J. R., HARWOOD-NASH, D. C., FITZ, C. R.: The neuroradiology of childhood choroid plexus neoplasms. Amer. J. Roentgenol. Radiol. Ther. Nucl. Med. **118**, 116—133 (1973)
20. WILLIAMS, B.: Is aqueduct stenosis a result of hydrocephalus. Brain **96**, 399—412 (1973)
21. WOOD, J. H., BARLET, D., JAMES, A. E., UDVARHE-LYI, G. B.: Normal pressure hydrocephalus. Diagnosis and patient selection for shunt surgery. Neurology **24**, 517—526 (1974)
22. YU, H. C., DECK, M. D. F.: The clivus deformity of the Arnold Chiari malformation. Radiology **101**, 613—615 (1971)

Subject Index

Pediatric Radiology

Subscription Information
1977: Volume 6 (4 issues)
Sample copies available upon request.

All countries (except North America)
DM 128,–, plus postage and handling.
Please order through your bookdealer
or directly with
Springer-Verlag
Promotion Department
Journals
Postfach 105280
D-6900 Heidelberg

North America:
US $ 55.40, including postage and
handling. Subscriptions are entered
with prepayment only. Please order
through your bookdealer or directly
with
Springer-Verlag New York Inc.,
175 Fifth Avenue, New York 10010
NY, USA

As a result of the rapid advances made in recent decades, pediatric radiology has
become a significant, independent, and clinically important speciality. In order
to fulfill the increasing need of child-health specialists for keeping fully abreast
with all major developments in this new field, Pediatric Radiology, the only
journal devoted exclusively to the various aspects of pediatric radiology, was
founded in 1973.

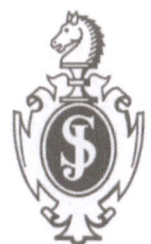

Springer-Verlag
Berlin
Heidelberg
New York

Pediatric Radiology publishes the following types of material:
1. Original papers report progress and results from all areas of pediatric
   radiology and its related fields.
2. Review articles and annotations reflect the present state of knowledge in
   special areas or summarize limited themes in which discussion has led to
   clearly defined conclusions.
3. Case reports of patients with rare and interesting diseases are presented. These
   case reports are primarily short descriptions directed to demonstrating one
   cardinal feature.
4. Technology, methodology, new apparatus, and auxiliary equipment together
   with modifications of standard techniques are discussed.
5. Pediatric Radiology presents a continuing statement of the world literature in
   pediatric radiology and related fields.

Ergebnisse der inneren Medizin und Kinderheilkunde

Advances in Internal Medicine and Pediatrics

Neue Folge

Herausgeber:
P. Frick, G.-A. von Harnack
G. A. Martini, A. Prader, R. Schoen,
H. P. Wolff

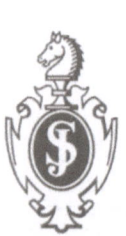

Springer-Verlag
Berlin
Heidelberg
New York

Band 32
36 Abbildungen. IV, 364 Seiten (101 Seiten in Englisch). 1972.
Gebunden DM 165,–; US $ 72.60
ISBN 3-540-05646-7
Die retroperitoneale Fibrose (Ormond'sche Krankheit). – Immun-pathogonese chronischentzündlicher Lebererkrankungen. – Enzymmuster am Nephron. Quantitative histochemische Ergeb-nisse. – The Systemic Mucopolysacharidoses.

Band 33
24 Abbildungen. IV, 333 Seiten (63 Seiten in Englisch). 1972.
Gebunden DM 165,–; US $ 72.60
ISBN 3-540-05883-4
Mißbildungen bei Zwillingen. – Zur Pathogenese der Arterios-klerose von Aorta und Extremitätenarterien. – Untersuchungen zur Klassifizierung akuter Leukämien. – Australia Antigen, an Antigen Associated with Viral Hepatitis. – Mineralocorticoid-syndrome. Calcium Absorption in Health and Disease.

Band 34
41 figures. IV, 237 pages (74 pages in German). 1974.
Cloth DM 124,–; US $ 54.60
ISBN 3-540-06519-9
Immunosuppressive Therapie. – Primary Reninism, A Surgically Curable Form of Hypertension. – Drug Selection and Dosage in Renal Isufficiency. – Calcium Metabolism and Kidney Disease. – Prä-, peri- und postanal bedingte Schwachsinnsformen.

Band 35
30 Abbildungen. IV, 206 Seiten. 1974.
Gebunden DM 98,–; US $ 43.20
ISBN 3-540-06781-7
Die primäre biliäre Cirrhose. – Hereditäre Enzymdefekte des Erythrocyten: Expressivität und molekulare Heterogenität ano-maler Enzymproteine. – Nephropathie durch Analgetica.

Band 36
44 Abbildungen, 5 Schemata. IV, 206 Seiten (18 Seiten in Englisch). 1974.
Gebunden DM 124,–; US $ 54.60
ISBN 3-540-06818-X
The Lung as a Chemical Filter. – Die chronische Polyarthritis. Veränderungen und konservative Behandlung.

Band 37
49 Abbildungen. IV, 222 Seiten (86 Seiten in Englisch). 1975
Gebunden DM 144,–; US $ 63.40
ISBN 3-540-07040-0
Disequilibrium Syndrome in Hemodialysis. – Kontrollierte Hyper-thyreosetherapie. – Radiusaplasie mit Thrombocytopenie. – Ein genetisches Syndrom. – Indications and Results of Coronary Bypass Surgery. – The Importance of Bile Acids in Human Diseases.

Band 38
34 Abbildungen, 34 Tabellen. IV, 232 Seiten (58 Seiten in Englisch). 1976.
Gebunden DM 124,–; US $ 54.60
ISBN 3-540-07640-9
Die internistische Therapie der malignen Lymphome. – Autosomal Chromosome Aberrations. – A Review of the Clinical Syndromes Caused by Structural Chromosome Aberrations, Mosaik-Trisomies 8 and 9, and Triploidy. – Alpha-1-Antitrypsin.

Preisänderungen vorbehalten